TOUR GUIDE

INSTRUCTION MANUAL FOR GROUPS OF ALL SIZES

Annette Reeder

designed publishing

Dear Tour Guides,

We are honored you have chosen to take into your hands this Leader Guide to a very exciting Bible study. Many Bible studies have effectively guided us on the road to gain understanding of Scripture. Now we are going to take that one step further and include our body's most precious necessity: food and its byproduct - health. For years Christ has been shared in various ways but now we have the gift of food to lead others to knowing Him in a new and refreshed way. Food truly is a gift, one that is meant for our nourishment but also as a tool to show the love and care of our Lord. Reaching others through the power of food is our mission. Thank you for joining us.

Seeing lives changed both physically and spiritually will be your reward for leading others on this journey. Reading this book along with doing the Bible study in advance will help you get a clear picture of all that is involved.

This class is not about what products to buy, even though suggestions are offered. Instead the underlying reason for our teaching is to show the participants that God loves them just as He does you, and that you are a special part of His plan. That plan requires treating our body as the gift it is. This means feeding it the foods required for health and caring for it with exercise and forgiveness. Please do not use this class as a platform to promote a personal business as this will distract from the Bible study.

As the leader you will be in a position to help many people come to know Christ in a real and personal way. Ask your pastor or ministry leader to review this material so he/she can be praying with you as you lead your group.

When you are ready to begin, let the office of Designed Healthy Living know so we can pray for you. Also check out the Designed Healthy Living Facebook page for posting fun notes about your class.

Most of all enjoy the study, have fun with your foodie friends, and share the love of Christ with all who attend. God has brought them to your class for a purpose and now you are their guide on this new food adventure.

May God richly bless you and your treasures class,

Annette Reeder and Dr. Dick Couey

Designed Healthy Living, 14172 Gordons Lane, Glen Allen, VA 23059.
www.designedhealthyliving.com
yourfriends@designedhealthyliving.com
804.798.6565

Printed in the USA

ISBN: 978-0-9853969-3-0

This Leader Guide is based on the book, Treasures of Healthy Living by Annette Reeder and Dr. Richard Couey. Published by Designed Publishing.

To the best of our knowledge the FDA has not read this Bible study nor approved it for church or personal use. If they did they may find the information against current policy. Therefore we are obligated to tell you the information contained in this Bible study guide is educational and merely offers nutritional support. It is not intended to replace medical advice. Seek a medical professional before making any changes to your diet or health program.

Table of Contents

Introduction for Treasure Hunt Guides

Welcome and thank you for your willingness to guide others on their treasure hunt towards healthy living. This manual will be your resource to facilitate a successful class and includes aids for a timeline for your meetings, review questions, extra talking points and worksheets. There are also resources online at www.designedhealthy-living.com. We continually update the website so check back often to see what is new. Feel free to contact the offices of Designed Healthy Living if you need assistance or additional suggestions.

OVERVIEW OF THE STUDY

To better understand God's love is paramount for this study. Otherwise, this would just be another health plan. In addition, *Treasures of Healthy Living Bible Study* gives a balanced approach to improving health and the understanding of God's provision. The study examines three principles related to food:

Principle 1: Eat only substances God created for food.

Principle 2: Eat the foods close to the way God designed, with very little alterations.

Principle 3: Don't let any food become your god.

RESOURCES REQUIRED

TREASURES OF HEALTHY LIVING BIBLE STUDY

This study is divided into 2 six-week parts, plus an introduction week and concludes with a banquet in the final week. The study is designed to be completed in 13 weeks, but can be divided into part I and part II offered at separate times. It can also be completed as an individual or family study.

- Each week includes four days of Bible study, personal application, and Foodie Fridays. Foodie Fridays are encouragements for participants to have a Foodie friend with whom to share their new food experiences.
- Action Plan: Each week participants are asked to write one goal on their Action Plan sheet in the back of the study. This is vital for their success to make small simple changes that will last a lifetime. When they have done this for 12 weeks their health will begin to reflect the value of God's Word. As leaders it is imperative you remind them weekly.

TREASURES OF HEALTH NUTRITION MANUAL

A resource you will not want each person to be without, this book will give more in-depth information on foods, vitamins and overall health for everyone in the family. Highlights for specific health topics needed to complete each week's lesson are found throughout this treasure. Each person must have a copy of this book.

HEALTHY TREASURES COOKBOOK

This collection of tasty recipes applies the three core principles and uses whole foods. It surely will become a keepsake as the participants learn about new foods. *Healthy Treasures* is highly recommended.

Treasures of Healthy Living DVD Series

A true treasure to add to this adventure. This set of 8 DVDs and 13 weeks of lessons along with extra bonus sessions is truly a gem to not miss on the journey. The teachings will greatly enhance each week's learning.

WEEKLY MEETINGS

Two-hour group meetings would include:

Prayer requests and praises

Video Intro for Today's Topic

Bible Study Review

Action Plan Review

Taste and See

Health Topic presentation on DVD

Meetings of either of one hour or 90 minutes can be effective. The key is careful planning. Facilitating this class during weekly lunches such as a business or Sunday evening class can be easily accomplished if one day is devoted to review and discussion and another day is for viewing the DVD. Another option is for each participant to purchase their own copy of the DVDs or CDs.

Video Intro for Today's Topic – Begin each class with a 2-4 minute introduction via the DVD's. This helps focus on the topic of the week and introduces simple application principles.

Bible Study Review - This time is crucial to the value of this study and for life-long application. Guard this step or the class becomes just another health class and another 'expert' will come along and distract from God's Truth. The truth of our health comes solely from God's Word so guard this time carefully.

Action Plan Review – At the end of each week's discussion of the Bible study participants need to create or share their action plan to reinforce their learning and application from each week's lesson. If time is short this may be covered on alternating weeks. The Action Plan is located on page 323 of the Bible Study.

Taste and See - This is a time for participants to experience healthy food and to share preparation tips with one another. The leader should bring Taste and See foods for the first three weeks. (Suggestions are found in each week's planning section.) Then participants will enjoy bringing Taste and See foods for the remaining weeks of the class.

As the leader, if you feel like this aspect of the class is too much of a burden, consider inviting someone to co-lead the class and handle this portion. Alternatively, you can ask someone to bring the food each week instead. It will make every week a foodie adventure.

Starting Week 4 the participants bring food. This food can be related to the week's topic or a food of their choice. A copy of the recipe should be brought for each participant unless the recipe is from the *Healthy Treasures Cookbook*. Encourage them to do both—using the cookbook as well as transforming their regular family recipes into a healthier variety. Ultimately they choose what they want to bring in. There will be recipe suggestions each week if needed.

Use these rules for class food: no restaurant or processed food including deli or food bars; no unhealthy ingredients including pork; no white flour or white sugar; nor white rice products. It may be necessary to provide utensils and plates or cups. Everyone in the class is required to bring in food even husbands and kids. Sometimes they have come up with the best delights!

For the final week a banquet allows all participants to bring a dish to share. Some classes invite spouses or church staff to join this event. A sign-up sheet for this event might include entrees, appetizers, bread, salads, vegetables, and desserts.

In Week 4 the topic is vegetables. The best way to enhance the material is to have ALL participants bring in an assigned food. A guide for organizing the food for this week is found on pages 29 & 33 in this Tour Guide. A print-out for the Fabulous Foodie Fun is in the appendix.

<u>Health Topic DVD</u> – Each topic is designed to enhance the weekly learning and application.

CLASS COST AND EXPENSES

The cost for participants depends on what is required of them. When Annette Reeder teaches the classes she charges for the Bible Study, Nutrition Manual, Cookbook, plus the cost for food. Typically $10 – 20 total per person will cover the cost of food for the first three weeks that the leader brings in food. The cookbook is greatly encouraged but can be optional. The class is more coherent if the leader follows the food ideas presented for each topic and has the participants pay that expense. If a husband and wife; or parent and child take the class, the fees for the books are for one set of 3. The second person pays only the food fee.

If the DVDs have not been purchased as an investment by the church or facilitator then the cost can be divided among the participants.

LEADER PREPARATION

Pray

Please enter into this time of preparation with a heart of prayer. Participants will view the leader as an example of healthy living both nutritionally and spiritually or as one who sincerely desires it. This is not to say that a leader has to be perfect. None of us are. But the leader should be striving toward better health. It would be wise to have a prayer partner while you lead this study.

Review

Be comfortable. Take the time to read through the whole study before teaching it to others for a better understanding of how the Bible and resources fit together. The more comfortable you are with the material, the more natural the information will flow. Make sure to preview each health topic segment prior to class.

Meeting Tips

- The health information in this study is probably new and participants will have lots of questions. Be prepared to provide answers or to give resources. Encourage participants to write down their concerns and so avoid having one person monopolize the class. As leader, feel free to submit those concerns and questions to yourfriends@designedhealthyliving.com. Our staff will try to return answers quickly.

- Always be respectful of people's time. They have joined this class with the assumption that it will start and end promptly. The best way to organize meeting time is to be familiar with the material and stay focused.

- The respect for time is also true when taking prayer requests. It may be helpful to guide the sharing of prayer requests. A guided question could be "In light of the health topic that we learned about last week, how can we pray for **you**?" Prayer time should stay focused on class members and not venture to all family members and coworkers, neighbors, etc. who have health problems. This class is for the nurturing of these attendees. There are other opportunities in church or in other groups to extend these prayer requests.

- As you reference Bible verses make sure to read from your Bible and not from the study. God's Word is always the authority.

- Add humor to the discussion. The study of food is a happy topic!

- Thank participants for their participation and comments.

Logistics

- Determine a location and time for the meetings. Keep in mind the number of participants you expect.

- Arrange for access to visual equipment for the weekly DVD. Make sure you know how to use all functions to properly operate the DVD and to pause it for reference. A marker board is also useful for particular weeks.

- Participants should be seated at tables and accommodations for those with physical disabilities should be available.

- Be mindful about holidays and weather issues that may occur during class dates. Have a plan for inclement weather cancellation. Notice that starting Week 7, participants are encouraged to participate in a "Daniel" fast (no meat or dairy) for 3 weeks. This may be very tricky if it occurs over holidays so consider starting the fast earlier than Week 7, if necessary.

- Keep a record of participants in order to follow up by phone or e-mail.

- Leaders may order all materials for the class or can require participants to order individually. If the leader places the order, make sure to keep a record of payments due. Church and group discounts are available from Designed Healthy Living.

For each meeting bring:

★ A smile on your face

★ A prayerful heart

★ Attendance sheet (your own design)

★ Individual info sheet (for the first meeting or any meeting with new participants – design your own to gather information regarding allergies and what they expect to get from the class.) optional.

★ Taste and See sign-up sheet for weeks 4 through 11 (Leader provides weeks 1-3)

★ Health Topic DVD

★ Study materials – printed Viewer Guide handouts (found in Appendix)Some leaders have these printed ahead of the class starting and put in a binder for each participant.

★ Bible

★ Filtered water

★ Cups/plates/napkins/utensils for serving and eating

★ Cleaning supplies so you can leave the meeting room neat.

Introduction
Are You Ready to Discover - Treasure of Health?

AGENDA

Welcome & Prayer

Introductions (20 minutes)

Video 1: Dr. Couey Introduction (4 minutes)

Video 1: Series Introduction (2 minutes)

Taste and See (15 minutes)

Video 2: Are You Ready to Discover the Treasure of Health? (38 minutes)

Discussion (20 minutes)

Wrap It Up (15 minutes)

BRING

- Carrot Cookies, Loaded Chocolate Oatmeal Cookies, and Calypso Fruit Salad
- Pure Water
- DVD 1
- Student Handouts – Viewer Guide: Are You Ready to Discover the Treasure of Health? (see Appendix)

WELCOME

Welcome participants and have them complete the Individual Information Sheet - optional.

PRAYER

Pray God will lead you all as you begin this hunt to understand God's love and His gift in this treasure of health.

INTRODUCTIONS

Introduce yourself and explain why you are leading the class.

Ask each participant to share their name and why they are taking the class.

VIDEO 1 & 2: Dr. Couey Introduction and Series Introduction

TASTE AND SEE

Share cookies you brought. The Calypso Fruit Salad can be made in front of the class to show ease of preparation.

Share: One of the benefits of this class is the opportunity to make and sample healthy food choices.

Explain: Taste and See

Each week we will taste samples of healthy foods. I will bring food the first 3 weeks and then each of you will have a chance to make a tasty and healthy recipe for us to try. You can bring in any food that is healthy according to the information we are learning in class. You should bring enough for everyone to have a sample, not a full meal. Also provide serving and eating utensils as needed. Lastly, bring copies of the recipe to share.

VIDEO 2:

"Are Your Ready to Discover the Treasures of Health?" Introduce video: *Annette Reeder is now going to share a little about this journey we are starting.*

♦ ♦ ♦

VIEWER GUIDE ANSWERS

Taste means: <u>to eat, to discover</u>

See means: to <u>observe, to experience</u>

Words that describe the health you desire: Individual answers.

PROVERBS 2:6

For the Lord gives <u>wisdom</u>; From His mouth comes <u>knowledge</u> and <u>understanding</u>.

PSALM 119:92-93

"If your law had not been my delight, then I would have perished in my affliction. I will <u>never</u> forget Your precepts, for by them you have <u>revived</u> me!"

PROVERBS 3:7-8

Do not be wise in your own eyes, fear the Lord and turn away from evil. It will be <u>healing</u> to your body and <u>refreshment</u> to your <u>bones</u>.

EXODUS 15:26

If you listen <u>carefully</u> to the voice of the Lord your God and <u>do</u> what is right in his eyes and <u>give ear</u> to His commandments, and <u>keep</u> all His statutes, I will put none of the diseases on you which I have put on the Egyptians, for I am the Lord <u>who heals you</u>.

DEUTERONOMY 4:39-40

Know therefore <u>today</u>, and take it to your heart that the Lord, <u>He is God</u> in heaven above and on the earth below; there is <u>no</u> other. So you shall keep His statutes and His commandments which I am giving you today that it may go well with you and with your <u>children</u> after you and that you may <u>live long on the land</u> which the Lord Your God is giving you for all time.

John Piper: What we <u>hunger</u> for, we <u>worship</u>.

◆ ◆ ◆

WRAP IT UP

Explain: Foodie Fridays and Foodie Friends

I am asking each of you to choose someone in your life (or someone in this class) that would be willing to be your Foodie Friend. Foodie Friends will join you in the hunt for good health by holding you accountable to what you are learning and by searching for and tasting new food ideas each week. (Suggestions: spouse, friend, older child, classmate)

HOMEWORK

Assignment for next week – Read the first chapter in the Bible study. This is a lengthy chapter but packed with lots of information. The other chapters are shorter.

Reading Assignment: *Treasures of Healthy Living* – Read "Introduction" page xv, "Starting the Treasure Hunt" page xvii, "Week 1: Treasure of Health" page 1.

In the *Treasures of Health Nutrition Manual* read "If Only I Had Known" page xiii, "Why Should Christians Be Healthy" page xv, "God Owns Our Bodies" page xvi, and "A Sample Day" page xix.

Health Assessment: On page 333 in the Bible Study is the Health Assessment. Take time this week to fill it out and date it. This will help you mark the changes in your health as you continue on this journey.

Action Plan: Each week you will be asked to record on page 323 one simple change you are willing to make so this journey can be rewarding for a lifetime. Small, simple changes last. Remember to do this and at the end of the study you will see how 12 small, simple changes add up to big transformations in your attitude and health.

Encourage each participant to press on – the rewards are coming!

CLOSE IN PRAYER.

Week One

Introduction—A Healthy Bank Account

AGENDA

Welcome & Prayer (10 minutes)

Video: Healthy Food Intro (5 minutes)

Review: Week 1 (pp. 1-6) (20 minutes)

Foodie Reports and Praise Tickles (10 minutes)

Taste and See (15 minutes)

Video: Healthy Bank Account (27 minutes)

Video (if time permits): Mindless Eating (23 minutes)

Wrap It Up

BRING

- Suggested Foods - Muesli Mix, Muffins – your choice,

- Ingredients to make smoothies in class: yogurt, frozen fruit, raw honey, protein and flax seeds.

- Keifer - Annette Reeder usually brings in Keifer in various flavors for them to try and then they can add granola in it or the muesli mix. This is a quick breakfast.

- See Taste and See for this week for any suggestions on other foods to bring.

- Sign-up Sheets- Bring sign-up sheets for participants to bring in food starting week 3- Grains.

- Vegetable Sign Up Sheet - Bring in a sign-up sheet for Week 4 Veggies when everyone brings in a vegetable or fruit.

- DVD 1

- Fresh Market Painting

WELCOME

Greet everyone and have newcomers fill out the Individual Information Sheet (sample in Appendix).

PRAYER

Ask each participant, if willing, to share one health goal they would like the group to pray for. They can also share their Action Plan step as a prayer request.

VIDEO – Healthy Food Choices Intro

REVIEW (questions are in bold and answers are in italics)

Read Proverbs 2:1-6

In your study you wrote down the three verbs. What were they? (p. 3)

1) *Receive my words*

   How do we do this? *Read the Bible*

2) *Treasure My commandments*

   How do we do this? *Guard them*

3) *Discover the knowledge*

   How do we do this? *By fellowshipping with Him we will discover knowledge. Fellowship with God is spending time with Him throughout our day.*

When you do these 3 things the verse goes on to tell you what God will give you. What are the blessings God will send? (p. 3)

Wisdom, knowledge and understanding

In today's society there is more information about health than ever in the history of this country. With all this information are we healthier than in past years?

No

Do you feel more or less confident in your ability to be healthy?

Own answers

What would improve your confidence?

From their reading participants should have learned their confidence comes from looking to Scripture. Help them pull this answer out if it does not come freely.

DISCUSS: Fulfillment – The study defined fulfillment as "a sense of achieving something expected, desired or promised." As we learn to trust God in this area of eating and health we will discover fulfillment.

Read John 10:10. How would fulfillment feel to you? (p. 5)

Own answers.

DISCUSS: John Jay, Christian Statesman 1799 (p. 12)

Some people want change without change. He refers to the Israelites complaining in Egypt then complaining on the way to the Promised Land. Many people prefer to remain in slavery.

Are you ready to leave the bondage of illness and chemicals?

Own answers.

What have you learned in the past that you need to leave behind?

Own answers.

What does the Promised Land, God's health, mean to you? How do you visualize it?

Own answers.

Ask someone to read Deuteronomy 4:39-40

What is your impression of this verse? What is God telling you? (p. 13)

Own answers

Reemphasize verse 40. *He asks us to keep His statutes and commandments and then it will go well with our children that we will live long on this land.*

TOOLS FOR THE JOURNEY (P.20)

Tool #1: Delight Yourself in the Law

Psalm 119- How many of you read this whole chapter? If you did then you read the longest chapter in the Bible. It is a chapter where the author is showing us how to delight in the law. From your answers, how does David describe the law of the Lord?

Perfect, restores the soul, makes wise the simple, right, pure, enlightening to the eyes, endures forever, righteous.

The lesson goes on to explain the different types of laws. This will help us know how to keep them.

What benefits spiritually, physically and emotionally did you discover from this chapter following the law?

Review some verses if you have time: verse 70-72, 89-91, 97, 98, and 99

Tool #2: The Three Principles (p. 24)

Review the three principles. What is an example of each principle?

1) <u>*Eat only substances God created for food. Avoid what is not designed for food.*</u> *Examples to avoid: processed cheese, potato chips, cool whip, imitation vanilla etc. Dairy is a food man alters greatly.*

2) <u>*As much as possible, eat foods as they were created-before they are changed or converted into something humans think might be better.*</u>
Example to include: grains, old fashioned oatmeal, nuts, seeds, real fruit instead of a fruit roll-up.

3) <u>*Avoid food addictions. Don't let any food become your god.*</u>*(yes, god is correct here)*
Example to avoid: caffeine

Tool #3: The Healthy Treasures Mediterranean Pyramid (p. 29)
Show Fresh Market Painting from Full Study Kit. More copies of this painting can be ordered from the Designed Healthy Living website. This painting gives an opportunity for families to discuss the treasures around the dinner table.

How does this pyramid look different from the way we currently eat?

Most people eat sweets as their main food group instead of the grains that should be our foundation.

What nuggets did you get from this week's lesson and how can you apply it?

Own answers.

FOODIE FRIEND

Please tell us who your Foodie Friend is and what you did together this week.

TASTE AND SEE

Serve the muffins, keifer and muesli mix and make smoothies in front of the class. Be creative with the smoothies. (You may want to bring smaller cups to make the creation serve more people.) Raw carrots and kale make a fun addition to the drinks. Grind up the whole flax seeds before adding the other ingredients for the smoothie. Refer to the *Nutrition Manual* for teaching helps for flax seeds, yogurt, osteoporosis and calcium. If you don't have time, assign these topics as a reading assignment for the coming week.

Always have pure water available with cups

Yogurt: Read the article about yogurt ahead of time. Review it with class. (If a question about probiotics comes up they can read more about that in the *Nutrition Manual*.) Bring samples of different kinds of yogurt.

Smoothies: A variety of fruits can be used in smoothies. Using a straw can sometimes encourage children to drink them. Some examples of good yogurts include Stoneyfield Farms (with 6 cultures) and Brown Cow (4 cultures). Beware of yogurt with Bovine growth hormones and sugar. Dannon and others lack quality cultures. If a sweetened yogurt is desired choose a fruit juice sweetened variety rather than the other sweeteners. Do NOT get aspartame or Splenda sweetened. You can add honey to plain yogurt for a tasty treat.

A recipe for a Green Smoothie can be found on the website under "Go for the Good" recipes. It has spinach in it and everyone is amazed at the good taste.

Yo-cheese: You can also drain plain yogurt in a yogurt funnel and make yogurt cheese. This can be substituted for mayonnaise, sour cream, or cream cheese. Show yogurt cheese maker and yogurt funnel if you have one. One cup of yogurt daily is recommended.

DISCUSS (If time allows)

Read ahead of the session the information in the *Nutrition Manual* - Osteoporosis and Calcium Magnesium. If there is time in the session today, lead a discussion on this important material.

VIDEO 1: "A Healthy Bank Account"

INTRODUCE: *Annette Reeder will show us how to balance this information we are learning while building our health.*

♦ ♦ ♦

VIEWER GUIDE ANSWERS

<u>Whole</u> foods build the <u>whole</u> body.

♦ Better Resistance to <u>Illness</u>

♦ Mental <u>alertness</u>

♦ Blood Sugar <u>stability</u>

♦ Great <u>attitude</u>

♦ Less or no <u>aches and pains</u>

♦ Energy and Flexibility (<u>mentally and physically</u>)

♦ Looking <u>good</u> Feeling <u>good</u>

Health Expenses:

<u>Fast Food</u> Diet

Sugar

Synthetic <u>Supplements</u>

Toxins

<u>Victim</u> Mentality

Lack of <u>Knowledge</u>

Dehydration

<u>Sporadic</u> Exercise

OTC and Rx <u>Medications</u>

Un-forgiveness

Stress

More health expenses than income = <u>Bankruptcy</u>

♦ ♦ ♦

VIDEO 2: If time permits show the "Mindless Eating" Video.

VIEWER GUIDE ANSWERS

• <u>Magazines</u>

• TV

• Your <u>Kitchen</u>

• Size of <u>servings</u> and Number of <u>servings</u>

• <u>Commercials</u>

• <u>Distractions</u>

• Size of <u>plates</u>

ARE YOU REALLY HUNGRY?

Physical Hunger

• Builds <u>gradually</u>

• Strikes <u>below</u> the neck

• Occurs <u>several</u> hours after a meal

• <u>Goes away</u> when full

• Eating leads to feelings of <u>satisfaction</u>

Cues to the good stuff

Be <u>happy</u>

Emotional Hunger

• Develops <u>suddenly</u>

• <u>Above</u> the neck

• Unrelated to <u>time</u>

• <u>Persists</u> despite fullness

• Eating leads to <u>guilt</u> and <u>shame</u>

Experience the <u>season</u>

Think 20%	Eat <u>slower</u>
Set a beautiful <u>table</u>	Minimize <u>temptations</u>
Be vigilant	Keep it simple
Keep your <u>perspective</u>	Give thanks
Watch yours and your spouse <u>expressions</u>	

You are the nutritional gatekeeper.

Gate keepers control <u>72%</u> of the food decisions of their children and spouse.

♦ ♦ ♦

WRAP IT UP

Remind participants to complete each day of the study and to review their Action Plan from this past week. The Action Plan is vital for their success. Emphasize this each week to make sure they know where it is located in the Bible study and its importance.

HOMEWORK

Read Week 2 in the Bible study. The reading will suggest "Digging Deeper" in the *Nutrition Manual*. A deeper knowledge base will be acquired by this additional reading.

Here are the page numbers in the *Nutrition Manual* to help find the topic: "10 Commandments of Good Hydration" page 9, "Fluoride" page 301, "Water" page 7, "Milk" page 12, "Resveratrol" page 40, "Aspartame" page 104, and "Tea" page 11.

NEXT WEEK'S TOPIC TEASER: *We will be studying beverages and your Foodie assignment involves water!*

CLOSE IN PRAYER.

Week Two
Beverages — It's A Radical Life!

AGENDA

> Welcome & Prayer (5 minutes)
>
> Prayer and Praise Tickles* (10 minutes)
>
> Review: previous week (10 minutes)
>
> Video: Water (3 minutes)
>
> Review: Water and Beverages (pp. 37-63) (10 minutes)
>
> Taste and See (15 minutes)
>
> Video: It's a Radical Life (34 minutes)
>
> Wrap It Up (10 minutes)

BRING

- Suggested Ideas
- Raw Milk sample – if you can find it
- Ingredients for Almond/Rice Milk or bring premade
- Water – add ice and mint; cucumber water or lemon balm
- Wild Rice Fruited Salad and Lentil Salad
- Pure Water
- DVD 2

WELCOME

PRAYER and PRAISE TICKLES

What are some specific prayer requests related to struggles implementing what you are learning in our study?

*Praise Tickles: These are praises that God has shown you personally through this study that you have been able to implement or think about this week?

REVIEW: Previous Health Topics

> **How many of you have made decisions based on your health bank account?**
>
> **Did your actions create a deposit or withdrawal?**
>
> **What do you think is the cost of one person dealing with cancer?**
>
> **How much should we have in our health bank account to help prevent an illness or disease?**
>
> > *The answers will vary but what we want them to see is to not get into the mindset of a 5-day work week:*

eat healthy for 5 days and then splurge for 2 days. This will never build a healthy bank account that can withstand the epidemics plaguing our country.

Encourage them to teach the bank account theory to their kids. It is a practical teaching tool.

What are the three principles? List food examples included in each principle? (Ask a different person each week to recite the three principles.)

1. *Eat only substances God created for food.*
2. *As much as possible, eat foods as they were created.*
3. *Avoid food addictions.*

What steps have you taken this week to be more aware of the foods you eat?

Own answers,

VIDEO: Water Intro

REVIEW: Water and Beverages

Treasure Clue. Proverbs 4:20-22. Read out loud from your Bible or choose someone to read it.

How does this verse fit with our journey?

Own answers.

These first 6 weeks we are going to fill our treasure chest with the greatest bounty God ever designed. Our journey begins with the first gift to put in our treasure chest – the gift of water.

How can we apply the study of water to our treasure chest both physically and spiritually? (pp. 38-39)

How do we know when we are thirsty spiritually and physically? (pp. 41-42)

Pull answers from their study questions. "Thirsty"

What similarities did you find between Jesus and water? (p. 39)

Jesus is perfectly designed – like water

Jesus satisfies - like water

How many of you calculated your water needs for the day? (p. 43)

Does this number surprise you?

What steps can you make to gradually build up to this amount?

Have them come up with specific plans to incorporate more water in their day.

How would you apply the three principles to water? (p. 44)

1. *Drink water since it was given to us by God.*

2. *Drink it purified without the additives and hype found in the stores such as vitamin water and other gimmicks.*

3. *Drink the right amount.*

What did you learn about milk? What surprised you? (pp. 45-51)

How do we apply the three principles to milk?

1. *Milk is given to us by God to drink.*

2. *Raw milk is closest to the way He designed it. All other milks have been altered. – So buy a cow!*

3. *Many people are addicted to dairy – particularly cheese. Dairy products can cause digestive problems.*

What factors do we need to keep in mind when it comes to consuming juice? (p. 52)

Too much sugar and lack of fiber

How do we apply the three principles to juice and wine? (p. 57)

1. *Juice is a drink made from foods given to us by God.*

2. *Juice freshly squeezed or pressed is close to the way God designed it. But juice in the stores is loaded with sugars and additives. Fresh pressed is best. Concentrates are the least nutritious. Kid's drinks typically have less than 10% juice and the rest is flavorings and sugar. It is best to dilute juice. Wine today is more addictive then in biblical days and it alters the senses.*

3. *Juice can be addictive to kids. Too much sugar. Wine causes a lot of problems in our society as listed in the study.*

Matthew 22:29 AMP: You are wrong because you know neither the Scriptures nor God's power.

How many times do we make choices because we are tired of trying to do the right thing? How many times do we just give up – even if only for a short time?

The first week of your study mentioned that those who give up on the treasure hunt too soon do not reap the whole blessing.

Applying these truths to beverages:

What is one reason not to drink diet soda? (p. 59)

Artificial sweeteners fool the brain cells by masking as sugar which affects liver function and eventually ends up causing us to feel false hunger.

Apply the three principles to the following drinks:

Soda, Gatorade, Propel, vitamin water, hot chocolate

The participants should be able to answer these questions by now. You may find it helpful to search the ingredients in these drinks. The result of your search may totally surprise you. Once you do this search you will never drink these again!

Name one benefit of green tea. (p. 59-60)

inhibits the growth of cancer cells, kills cancer cells without harming healthy tissue, lowers ldl cholesterol, inhibits the abnormal formation of blood clots

ACTION PLAN

Take time today to be sure the participants are marking their Action Plan Sheet regularly. Suggestions for beverages on the Action Plan would include: adding water to their day until they reach the recommended amount of ½ their body weight in ounces, gradually going off soda, switching to a green tea, or even just measuring out the right amount of water to see how much it looks like.

Any step forward is a good step. Help them come up with one action plan step to take. It can be simple or complex but simpler is better.

FOODIE FRIEND

Who is your foodie friend? What have you and your foodie friend discovered? Have you taken trips to the store together, shared recipes, shared thoughts, etc.? Your foodie friend will help you stay on track and make great discoveries.

TASTE AND SEE

Let the class sample the different milk varieties you brought in such as almond milk, raw milk or even soy milk. Soy milk must be organic and state non-GMO on the label. (Read about this in the *Nutrition Manual.*)

Serve the foods you brought in: Wild Rice Fruited Salad and Lentil Salad

Grocery Tips: Water - don't be fooled by marketing or hype.
- Filter your own water at home: economical and a good filter removes lead plus other harmful contaminants.
- Flavored water is not a good choice.
- Tea and coffee – organic is the better choice.
- Juice – buy organic, fresh pressed is the highest quality but hard to find and costly. It is best to make your own with a juicer. If buying organic juice, dilute with 50% water to be economical and less sugar per serving.

Try making your own juice with a professional juicer – the taste is amazing. The Vita Mix machine makes a great smoothie. You will find a link to the Vita Mix on the Designed Healthy Living website and all purchases of products from the Designed Healthy Living website allow us to use the profits to benefit the military and missionaries. We offer our resources; books, DVDs and other products at greatly reduced rates so they can stay on mission. By supporting us with the purchase of these products you help make this possible.

◆ ◆ ◆

VIDEO: It's a Radical Life

VIEWER GUIDE ANSWERS

All living things begin as a <u>cell</u>.
 A group of cells create a type of <u>tissue</u>.
  A group of tissues create a particular <u>organ</u>
   A group of organs create an <u>organ system</u>.
    A group of organ systems create an organism.   Like You ☺.
       Everything that happens in the body happens at the <u>Cellular Level</u>.
The human body has 11 organ systems, see how many you can name:

Digestive, cardiovascular, respiratory, integumentary (skin), skeletal, muscular, nervous, endocrine (hormones), lymphatic, urinary and reproductive.

Basic Needs of a Cell:
 ◆ Water
 ◆ Oxygen
 ◆ Protein
 ◆ Food

Each person's responsibility:
 1. Supply <u>good food</u>
 2. Avoid <u>toxins</u>

Are they all Bad?   **NO** The Answer to Free Radical Damage: <u>Antioxidants</u>
Antioxidants are God's gift for free radical "damage control".
 1. Provide the extra <u>electron</u>.
 2. Provide a <u>protective</u> shield.
 3. <u>Disarms</u> the free radical.
How many antioxidants do we require? *Depends on each person and their exposure to free radicals.*

◆ ◆ ◆

WRAP IT UP

As you go through the week, see if you notice sources of free radicals in your environment or food. Think about ways to eliminate them.

HOMEWORK:

Read Week 3(Grains) in study. Have them sign up to bring in food each week and start the sign up for Week 4, fruits and vegetables. Remind them to fill out the Action Plan Sheet and commit to try one recipe from the *Healthy Treasures Cookbook.*

CLOSE IN PRAYER.

Week Three
Grains — Divine Design in Digestion

AGENDA

> Welcome (5 minutes)
>
> Prayer and Praise Tickles (10 minutes)
>
> Review: Previous weeks (20 minutes)
>
> Video: Grains Introduction (2 minutes)
>
> Review Week 3 Lesson (pp. 65-90)
>
> Taste and See
>
> Video: Divine Design in Digestion (35 minutes)
>
> Wrap It Up

BRING

- Food - The participants should be bringing in food now but if you want to continue to contribute, we suggest the Barley Cakes and the Unleavened Bread (with Olive Oil Dipping Sauce).
- Grains – if you have a supply of grains or can purchase some at the store this would be beneficial for students to see. Typical grains found in local stores: oatmeal, brown rice, couscous and popcorn; in better stores: wheat, spelt, kamut, amaranth, millet, and quinoa.
- DVD 2

WELCOME

Open by reading John 6:47 *I tell you the truth; he who believes has everlasting life. I am the bread of life.*

Since Genesis, God has provided us with bread and supplied the idea of its full benefit to physical life. Jesus refers to Himself as bread and therefore we know that God has supplied us with the answer to having an eternal life.

PRAYER and PRAISE TICKLES

Praise Tickles - ways God is working in your life or your family's life because of this study.

Prayer requests concerning struggles with implementing these new health ideas?

REVIEW - Previous week's lessons

> **Share how you are making deposits into your bank account and what benefits you are seeing.**
>
> **What are two antioxidants that are needed every day to help avoid free radical damage?**
> *Vitamin E and C*

How many of you were aware of the number of glasses of water you were drinking this week?

What have you noticed physically (except for increased trips to the bathroom) with this change?

Many times it will increase fullness, allow you to eat less, and help skin feel more supple.

How did you try to add yogurt into your diet this week? Did it bring about any physical benefits that you were able to notice?

What is one benefit of calcium?

Strengthens bones, aids in muscle relaxation and contraction, lowers blood pressure, and reduces PMS symptoms.

VIDEO: Grains Introduction

REVIEW: Grains Lesson (pp. 65-90)

Grains are used throughout Scripture – let's look at the symbols of life that you read about in Scripture. (pp. 66-71)

Genesis (p. 67) and the story of Isaac: How large was the harvest reaped? What do you think this is a symbol of?

Hundredfold, symbol of blessing, God the Provider

Deuteronomy 8:1-11: What is God teaching us in this passage?

If we follow His commands He will provide for our needs.

What grains does the Promised Land contain?

Wheat, barley

In the story of Ruth what symbols did you see?

God the Provider, Symbol of Redemption, Symbol of Fellowship

In Ezekiel we read about instructing a prophet. What symbol do you see here?

God the Provider

1 Samuel: What symbol is shown when David took food to his brothers who were fighting the Philistines?

Blessing, Unity, Fellowship

What is the symbol of grain when Abigail takes food as a peace offering?

Forgiveness, Redemption, Unity

Psalm 4:7: What is the symbol here?

God the Provider – God's presence is all that is needed to sustain life.

Matthew 12:1: What is the symbol?

God the Provider, Blessing, Fellowship

Matthew 14:13-21: How many were fed with five loaves of bread? What are the symbols?

5 loaves fed 5,000 men plus women and children with 12 baskets left over. Shows fellowship and God as the provider

Matthew 26:26: As Jesus broke the bread, what did it symbolize?

His Body – Provision, Redemption

What is the symbol of grain in Acts 2?

Unity and Fellowship

QUESTIONS FOR DEEPER UNDERSTANDING AND APPLYING THE SPIRITUAL TRUTHS OF BREAD

From these symbols of life which include forgiveness, God the Provider, gladness, redemption, blessing, unity and fellowship – do you think bread was important in biblical days?

Is it important to us today?

Scripture instructs us to teach our children and grandchildren what God has taught us. Could these truths be shared around the dinner table?

How do grains prove there is a Creator? (pp. 71-72) See Bible study for these answers.

Do you think fiber is very important in our diet? Why? (pp. 73-74)

More energy, weight control, aids in prevention of disease

Let's look at how you planned a diet to get 35 grams of fiber in your diet. (pp. 74-75)
Write this out on a board as they mention foods. List the grams of fiber and how many servings are needed to obtain the total amount of fiber. If the list is well planned it should show that it is not hard to get the daily amount of fiber needed.

We learned in our previous lessons that Vitamin E is very important for what process?

Getting rid of free radicals

What food will give us a good supply of vitamin E without the need of supplements?

Bread – whole grains

The fiber in bread will also increase our body's ability to make vitamin B. This is another benefit of making your own bread from freshly milled flour.

Many people are concerned with eating bread and weight gain. The fiber in whole grains is designed to give us fullness before we can overeat and get fat. Making your own fresh milled bread will give you these nutrients.

Show types of whole grains as discussed on pages 78-79 in the study.

Show the different grains you were able to find at the local stores. Discuss how to use them and typical recipes they could be used in. Grain recipes found in the *Healthy Treasures Cookbook* include: grain, barley, breads, kamut, couscous, quinoa, oats, wild rice, spelt and wheat.

Isaiah 55:2 (p. 84) Have someone read this verse aloud.

How can we relate to this verse with what we have learned from this chapter on grains? *Own answers*

How can we rephrase this verse as a prayer to God?

For years we have spent our money on what we thought was bread but now we learn that it was not the wholesome food God designed for our bodies. Because of this purchase our body was not satisfied. Our wages were wasted. But then the verse goes on to say "Listen ... eat what is good. Delight in abundance." The bread God designed is good and it will bring abundance in our health and overall we-being.

How do we apply the three principles to grains? (p. 88)

TASTE AND SEE:

Encourage the participants to explain their food dish and describe the ingredients they used. Have them share if they had to search and find a new food for the recipe and where it was located. The food brought in is not intended to feed a hungry crowd but just provide tasting samples. If the church or home does not supply utensils for the food then the person bringing in the food will need to supply them. This is different from earlier suggestions.

Grocery Tips:

Whole grains can be found in a typical grocery store but it is best not to depend on marketing to lead you to believe what is a true whole grain.

Oatmeal in the least processed form is steel cut oats. Some class members have even found oat groats which is just the oat in the natural form and uncut. It tastes really good when cooked like oatmeal. Beans, legumes, flax seed, and other whole grains are in regular stores.

Bread – if it can sit on the shelf for more than 3 days from the date it was baked, it is processed beyond your health benefit. There is no better bread then what you make yourself as you mill your own fresh wheat and bake it yourself. Until then purchasing bread in the freezer section, such as Ezekiel Bread would be a good choice.

Schedule time now for your class to host a bread making class with a proficient bread maker or view the bread making DVD included with this set. The same 30 minute video can also be viewed from the website under Bread Baking at its Best.

VIDEO: Divine Design in Digestion

◆ ◆ ◆

VIEWER GUIDE ANSWERS

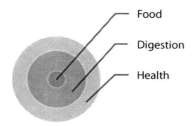

Our food choices are <u>connected</u> to our health.

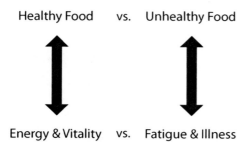

The digestive process is the center for <u>life</u> and <u>vitality</u>.

Elimination should happen <u>2-3</u> times per day.

To feel our best we must <u>digest</u>.

<u>Poor food</u> choices

<u>Lack of</u> fiber

Too much <u>stress</u>

<u>Toxic</u> environment

The digestive tract can heal itself in 3-5 <u>days</u>.

Constipation

The number one reason for constipation is lack of <u>fiber</u>.

We need <u>30-40</u> grams of fiber per day.

If fiber is not there to take out the toxins the body sends them to the <u>immune</u> system.

Functions of the Immune System

Protects, Repairs and <u>Prevents</u> Disease

1. <u>Water</u> & <u>fiber</u>
2. <u>Probiotics</u>

    These enhance the body's ability to absorb nutrition and help maintain a healthy intestine.
3. <u>Reduce</u> Stress

    Foods with a calming effect include herb teas, like chamomile. Deep breathing, exercise and relaxing activities help restore balance, peace of mind and joy for living.
4. <u>Provide and Protect</u> Enzymes and Vitamins

    Best source for enzymes are raw fruits and vegetables.
5. <u>Resist</u> Late Night and Overeating

    Our food choices are not just a <u>physical</u> matter but a <u>spiritual</u> matter also.

◆ ◆ ◆

WRAP IT UP

Encourage the class members to read about grains, fiber, leaky gut, and digestion in the *Nutrition Manual* pages 181-209. This will help them better understand these topics. Leaky Gut is unfamiliar to most people but experienced by many.

Schedule a bread making class either by watching the video (Bonus video included or on website) or host the class yourself. Contact Designed Healthy Living for tips on conducting this class, supplies needed and teaching notes. Annette Reeder can be scheduled to teach the class for your group if you want a true fun foodie experience. Her classes usually run 2 – 3 hours long and the group gets to experience 8 different recipes for making bread. The teaching starts with milling wheat and ends with sampling everything hot from the oven. A foodie's delight!

HOMEWORK

Encourage them to read Week 4 Fruits and Vegetables, try one new recipe from the *Healthy Treasures Cookbook*, and find the assigned vegetable to bring to class next week.

NEXT WEEK'S TASTE AND SEE:

Next week you will be looking at a variety of different veggies and fruit.

Make sure everyone is assigned a raw food to bring in from the list below. The food should be peeled and shredded or chopped as noted.

Here are some suggestions:

Turnip (shredded), **Sweet Potatoes** (shredded), **Beets**(raw shredded), **Parsnips** (shredded), **Jicama** (shredded), **Kohlrabi** (sliced finely), **Fennel** (sliced finely), **Leeks** (sliced finely), and **Rutabaga** (shredded). Celery root (shredded), Apples (chopped), Pears (chopped – look for new varieties), Plums (sliced), Peaches (sliced), Apricots, Berries, Cherries, Rhubarb (sliced) or Figs(sliced), Cabbage (chopped), and Carrots (shredded).

The first 9 ingredients are the most important. Make sure these are assigned first and reiterate the importance of bringing them in. If you have more people in class than the 9 , have the other sign up for others or have some bring in currants, coconut, and nuts. Next week have them taste these foods and then toss the **bold** foods together into a slaw. The dressing will need to be made ahead of time by you. If you have a small class the foods in bold print are the most important. The others are just for samples.

CLOSE IN PRAYER.

Week Four
Vegetables & Fruits — Go For the Good

AGENDA

Welcome (5 minutes)

Prayer and Praise Tickles (10 minutes)

Review: Previous 4 weeks (20 minutes)

Video: Vegetables Intro (3:20 minutes)

Review: Vegetables and Fruits (30 minutes)

Taste and See (20 minutes)

Video: Go For the Good (30 minutes)

Wrap It Up

BRING

- Bring a large bowl to mix the salad from all the vegetables being brought in to class.
- DVD 3

WELCOME

PRAYER AND PRAISE TICKLES

Ask questions to get your class thinking and responding. Try to balance more praise reports than prayer requests. Lead the opening prayer or ask someone else to pray.

REVIEW: Previous 4 Weeks

Are all free radicals bad?

No, they are made to destroy a virus or make hormones

What choices have you made to add to your and your family's bank account?

How have you made changes to switch from mindless eating to mindful eating?

What steps are you taking to improve yours or your family's digestion?

If you had to sum up the digestive tract in one word what would it be?

If they are not able to do so, let them sum it up in one sentence. Suggestions: The key to health. The beginning of happiness.

What types of whole grains did you add to your diet these past couple weeks?

Help them feel good about the positive changes they are making. Encourage those who are struggling with these food changes.

End each segment of the class on a positive note and with encouragement. Each person is dealing with unique health problems and social issues. This is to be a fun and supportive time. Depending on their food addictions this may be easy or hard. We have to meet them where they are and help them make small changes.

VIDEO: Vegetables Intro

REVIEW: Vegetables and Fruits

Have someone read Genesis 1:29 and Revelation 22:2

What conclusion might you reach by comparing these two verses and their locations in the Bible? (p. 93)

From the beginning of scripture in Genesis till the end of scripture in Revelation God is consistently offering the gift of healing. He offers it to us in the beginning for food and then in the end for healing. God loves everyone this much.

When you listed the vegetables you ate in the last 3 days, how well did you do? (p. 94) How about fruits? (p. 94)

Depending on their answers either congratulate them for a job well done or ask what they would like to add into their diets.

Review: Cruciferous vegetables: definition and different vegetables included. (p. 95)

How many do you typically get in your diet each week?

Are you willing to try some new ones?

Discuss: Daniel and its relevance to health today. Have them open their Bibles to Daniel 1.

Review verse 8: What two things did Daniel do in this verse? (p. 97)

1. *Daniel made up his mind or set his heart.*
2. *He asked permission of the commander of the officials to abstain from certain foods*

Part of God's character is to bring honor and glory to Him. This often occurs when one of God's children follows His directions or His will. How do Daniel's actions show his desire to do God's will?

He was intentional in all his actions – including the food he ate. He wanted every part of his life to be glorifying to the Lord.

When we are asked to do something against God's commands what should be our response? Should we ask permission? Is this a way for God to show you He is a mighty warrior going ahead of you in your defense?

Own answers.

Review verse 9: How did God intervene on Daniel's behalf?

see bible study for answers.

What happened after 3 years of following God's plan?

Daniel and his friends were smarter and healthier than all the other youths who had followed the king's special diet.

How would this translate in your life?

Own answers

See the Bible study for answers to the following questions.

Under "Your Health Is Worth It" on page 99, what did you learn about the benefit of fruits and vegetables and the 3 major health problems – obesity, heart disease, and cancer? (pp. 99-101)

Your lesson reviewed the difference between conventional farming and organic. What did you learn from this information? (pp. 104-106)

How can we apply what we learned to our food choices today?

How can we apply Proverbs 14:12 to what we are learning? (p. 106)

The way that seemed right to us for so long has lead us to sickness. Now we are learning the truth and with it comes life.

How can you apply the spiritual analogy for fruits to what you have learned? (pp. 109-110)

How can we apply the Three Principles to fruits and vegetables? (p. 113)

TASTE AND SEE:

Take the shredded vegetables that were written in bold print in last week's assignment and put them in nine individual bowls marked with numbers 1 – 9. Do not label the bowl with the name of the vegetable. Then have an answer key with the names of the vegetable corresponding to the bowl number. Have the participants take a piece of paper and number it 1-9 and then go around the tables taking small samples of each food. On their paper they need to write down their answer to each corresponding food. When everyone has had a chance to sample the vegetable varieties, toss the remaining vegetables into a slaw. Fennel and leeks may be too strong for this slaw so you might want to leave these out. A mixture of the sweet potato, beets, turnips, parsnips, rutabaga, and kohlrabi makes a perfect blend of flavors. Next add the currants, coconut and nuts. Toss this with a salad dressing and serve.

Suggested salad dressing: Fall Harvest Salad page 153 in the *Healthy Treasures Cookbook.*
Most of the time this is a big hit and a surprise to their taste buds at how good these particular foods taste raw.

◆ ◆ ◆

VIDEO: Go For the Good
Today our video will show fruits and vegetables, seasonal and farmers markets, and how to shop the grocery store produce aisle.

VIEWER GUIDE ANSWERS
God saw <u>all</u> that He had made and behold it was <u>very good</u>.
Good: <u>Excellent of its kind.</u>

◆ ◆ ◆

WRAP IT UP
Encourage them to try new fruits and vegetables.

HOMEWORK:
Read Week 5 – Herbs- in the Bible study. See how many resources you can find for herbs and vinegars. Experiment with herbs and vinegars this week. Replace fresh herbs for dry spices in a recipe. Remind the person who volunteered to bring food next week.

CLOSE IN PRAYER.

Week Five
Herbs — Making Melody with Your Heart

AGENDA

Welcome (5 minutes)

Prayer and Praise Tickles (10 minutes)

Review: Previous lessons

Video: Herbs Intro (2:40 minutes)

Review: Herbs (20 minutes)

Taste and See

Video: Making Melody with Your Heart (60 minutes)

Wrap It Up

BRING

- Garlic – whole raw
- Suggested food to bring in or make in class: Mexican Frito Salad, Bean and Corn Salsa, Cranberry/Feta/ Spinach Salad with Oriental Orange Dressing
- DVD 3
- Herb Guide and Chef's Companion – laminated cooking guides from the website or Full Study Kit

WELCOME

PRAYER and PRAISE TICKLES

Open with prayer and a Bible verse that you found particularly meaningful this week.

REVIEW: **What are some new foods your family has tried in these last weeks?**

What are some foods you have eliminated in your homes?

What is one thing you can do to assist your digestive tract in its daily job?

Fast, eat raw foods for enzymes, take an enzyme product, probiotics, and add fiber,
Flora – probiotics and mucosal lining which means no inflammation – This point may not have
been clearly understood from the digestion talk but you can add this as a teaching point.

How many days does it take for the digestive tract to heal itself?

3-5 days

What are some activities you and your foodie friend have participated in? What cooking experiences can you share with us?

VIDEO: Herb Intro

REVIEW: Herbs

In the King James Version of the Bible, herbs are mentioned four times in the first chapter of Genesis. Surely they have some significance. The first two references are cited in the account of Creation. Would someone read Genesis 1:11-12 (preferably KJV)?

The fact that each plant produces after its kind indicates that these plants are similar today to the way they were when first designed. The variation we see does not represent changes in the DNA or genetic code. Variation shows the tremendous latitude the original design had.

After God created man, He said:

> *Behold, I have given you every herb bearing seed, which is upon the face of all the earth, and every tree, in which is the fruits of a tree yielding seed; to you it shall be for meat. And to every beast of the earth and to every fowl of the air, and to everything that creepeth up on the earth, wherein there is a life. I have given every green herb for meat; and it was so. Genesis 1: 29-30 KJV*

The Bible mentions more than 120 kinds of plants. Some of these words, such as flowers, grains and nuts are used generically, without a specific kind being described. Other plant names, such as flax or onions are very specific. Biblical scholars and botanists are still not 100 percent sure what plants today correlate with all the biblical names.

What herbs did you know were in the Bible before you read this lesson? (pp. 118-199)

What herbs do you use in your cooking today?

> *Own answers – could include cinnamon, oregano, etc.*

What herbs do you use for medicinal purposes today or have used in the past?

> *Own answers – could include aloe.*

Your lesson went over various herbs in the Bible. The first ones were frankincense, myrrh, aloe, gall and mustard. **What did you learn about these herbs?** (pp. 118-119)

You went on to learn about coriander, garlic, hyssop, saffron, wormwood and cinnamon. (pp. 120-121)

How many of you have read in the Treasures of Health Nutrition Manual about garlic and its many uses in relieving health problems?

> *Go over some garlic remedies.*
> *Demonstrate: Garlic between the toes, in the ear, and anywhere that has an infection.*
> Passover (p. 122)

What was the purpose of bitter herbs during the Passover?

Affliction of slavery

What can we learn from the Passover? How can we use foods to teach our kids God's truths?

If we pass on to our children the story of God's deliverance from Egypt this will be a truth they can learn from. Using bitter herbs such as horseradish could be used as part of this teaching point. When we eat the bitter herbs it can remind us of the bondage we can find ourselves in and yet God delivered the Israelites and He will deliver us to. Food is the perfect tool to teach God's grace.

<u>Taking this treasure to heart:</u> **What truths have you learned regarding herbs that you would like to plant in your mind to treasure them always?** (p. 122)

What is one action step you can do with your knowledge of herbs? (p. 122)

Do you have any questions regarding standardized herbs? (p. 124)

(See study for answers)

How do we apply the three principles to herbs? (p. 127)

Principle 1 – Did God call herbs food for us? *Yes*

Principle 2 – Are they as close to the way He designed them as possible?

Some of them are when we eat them fresh from the garden or purchased fresh. Even some dried spices are close to the way God designed them. But some of the spices purchased in the store can be combined with other chemicals such as MSG, heavy metals or GMO plants. This means organic would be a better choice.

Principle 3 – Addictions

It is rare to have an herb addiction – but you never know!

Show the class the Herb Guide and Chef's guide. These guides make it simple and fun to add herbs in everyday recipes. These can be ordered from the website individually or in bulk.

What did you learn about salt, soy sauce, and MSG? (pp. 129-132) We will cover this in more detail in a later chapter.

TASTE AND SEE

These suggestions are perfect for taste and see time today.

- Making salads in class. Before class it is best to chop and assemble the ingredients in separate containers. Wash the lettuce thoroughly before taking to class.

SUGGESTED RECIPES:

Mexican Frito Salad

Bean and Corn Salsa

Cranberry, Feta, Spinach Salad with Oriental Orange Dressing.

Explanation: Describe the ingredients you are using in the salads and the health benefits of each one. If you are not certain about the health benefits, read about the ingredients in the *Treasure of Health Nutrition Manual*. Explain the health benefits of homemade dressing. Most store brand dressings have preservatives, MSG and artificial colorings. When making your own salad dressing it is best to use it within a couple weeks.

VIDEO: "Making Melody with Our Heart"

VIEWER GUIDE ANSWERS
Have the Nutrition Manual open to page 234-235 for this session.

◆ ◆ ◆

CPR - Care, Protect and Revitalize
Let's dare to be different
40% of those who suffer a heart attack never live to tell about it.
Diet – body needs healthy fat. – Olive Oil (page 76 in *Nutrition Manual*)
Good fats are very necessary.
Some fats heal and others kill

◆ ◆ ◆

WRAP IT UP:
Action Plan: *Looking at your action plan for the past several weeks. How many of you have accomplished some of your action plans?* Help them come up with simple action steps so they can have this accomplishment. Some people are ready for more complex steps in their journey, encourage both.

Further reading on this subject; 233-241 in the *Nutrition Manual*.

HOMEWORK – Read Week 6 in the Bible study, try one new recipe in the *Healthy Treasures Cookbook* and ask them to be open minded about this next chapter.

TOPIC TEASER FOR NEXT WEEK
Next week we will learn *What's For Dinner?* and how to get the right amount of protein in our diet and the health topic from Dr. Couey: *Inflammation.*

CLOSE IN PRAYER.

Week Six
Meat — We Have a Problem: Inflammation

AGENDA

Welcome

Prayer and Praise Tickles

Review: previous weeks (10 minutes)

Video: Meat Intro (3:20 Minutes)

Review: Meat and Protein

Taste and See (15 minutes)

Video: Dr. Couey: Controlling Inflammation & the Couey 6-Week Challenge
(40 minutes)

Conclusion to Part I video (4 minutes)

Wrap It Up

BRING

- Suggested recipes: Tortilla Bean Casserole, Nacho Casserole, Salsa Mini Meatloaves or other Enticing Entrée.
- DVD 4

WELCOME

PRAYER and PRAISE TICKLES

REVIEW previous weeks:

ACTION PLAN: This is a good time to review their steps to success on the Action Plan.

Who can recite the three principles?

Choose someone who has not done this before in class.

Last week, what did we learn from Exodus 15:26?

If they don't remember then let someone look it up.

Can anyone remember Hosea 4:6? If yes, recite and/or share the basic concept.

What other verses have made an impact in your study these past 6 weeks?

What steps are you taking to prevent free radicals?

Possible answers might be taking an all-natural vitamin E supplement, adding fresh milled bread into the diet, avoiding products that cause free radicals.

What steps are you taking to improve your digestive tract?

Answers might include – adding more whole grains, drinking more water, eating less, eating less often, more fiber, etc.

What steps are you taking to improve your cardiovascular system/ heart?

Answers might include adding healthy fats in the diet – olive oil, flax seeds, exercising, studying Gods word, eliminating stress, etc.

VIDEO: Meat Intro

REVIEW: Meat and Protein

How do we determine our focus and desire? (pp. 143-144)

See Bible study for answers. Without a desire for obedience to God then we will get caught up in the culture of what we can and cannot eat. Even the Christian culture will give you any answer you want.

Share: This Bible study is for those who are truly seeking to focus on foods given to us by God. These foods are listed in our owner's manual (Bible) and will bring years of good health and the energy to follow through with God's will. Many people are living and serving God in other areas but are not ready to focus on the foods they eat. Sometimes this is because of rebellion, laziness but other times it is just a lack of knowledge. (Lack of Discipline)

The good news is that God is bringing our current food crisis to the forefront with various epidemics of disease and He is showing us the news that the right foods bring health. Repeatedly whole foods in their natural state are making headlines with their health-promoting properties. If we had read our treasure map for health years ago, then this would have been no surprise.

Reflect on John Piper's poem and the question: (p. 143)

Have you ever considered desiring Him in your eating?

According to Deuteronomy 5:29, Why did God give us the Old Testament Law?

For guidance, 'that it may go well with them', and the obedience will be transferred to their kids and grandkids.

Read Psalm 19:7-11. (p. 145)

What benefit is there to keep the law?

Answers might include: it is perfect, restores the soul, make wise the simple, gives rejoicing, enlightening to the eyes, clean, more desirable than gold, great reward, sweeter than honey.

Read: Romans 14

Share: Eating meat was as confusing to these early Christians as it is to Christians today. Paul concluded that eating meat or not eating meat is not a basic tenet of Christianity. Eating the right kind of meat is not discussed in these verses. The argument is about clean meats some Christians considered to be defiled because it had been offered to idols. Early Christians observed the biblical distinction between clean and unclean meats until well after 70 AD. Romans was written in approximately 58 AD.

Should eating meat be an important issue?

Yes and no. According to the scriptures you read meat is important to our health and it can be a stumbling block to others, but it is NOT important for our salvation. It was important enough for God to give us clear directions. Remember He designed us and gave us the very best to eat. We keep settling for less. It is important to understand we have been set apart – clean meats are less toxic, less harmful.

When did God give us the option of eating meat?

After the flood; God has definitely given us meat to eat. Jesus ate meat. After the resurrection, Jesus cooked fish for the disciples on the beach.

Have everyone turn to Leviticus 11.

Share: These are laws God gave His people. Jesus is the fulfillment of the law. Jesus is the fulfillment of the sacrifices for our sins. No longer do we need a priest to intercede for us. Jesus is now our High Priest. When Jesus died on the cross, the curtain was ripped in two, from top to bottom, so that we can now have direct access to the Father. No longer do we have to go through the ceremonial law to get to the Father. His desire for all is to be reconciled to him through Jesus. (You have not been capitalizing the pronouns related to divinity.)

Some people believe Jesus is the fulfillment of all Law. Some think that dietary law should be looked into for the health of our vessel, but it makes no difference in your salvation whether you eat clean or unclean meat. Dietary law was given by a loving God who cares about our bodies, so that's why we should consider it, for the health of our vessels, created by him.

Are you ready to review the law regarding food?

Your lesson asked you to write out Lev. 11:44a. (p. 146)

What is God telling us in these verses?

To set ourselves apart and follow His leading.

Why would God ask us to be holy in the middle of a list of foods?

He is calling us to be different; to be like Him.

What is the requirement for an animal to be considered clean? (p. 147)

Divided hoof and chews the cud

What is the requirement for water animals to be clean?

Fins and scales

What is required of insects?

Winged, walk on all fours, jointed legs

Which foods surprise you?

Own answers

Read: Leviticus 11:11, 12, and 13.

The NASB uses the words abhorrent three different times. Each time it refers to the different food groups that were just outlined as clean and unclean. When He reflects back to the unclean he uses a very strong word – abhorrent. Some translations use the word abomination. These strong words give a strong message. He meant what he said. Since He used such strong language to describe these food groups, maybe we should pay attention to them. What do you think?

Read: Isaiah 65:2-5

How would you summarize this verse?

Do you as parents sometimes feel that you have done everything to instruct your kids in what is right but yet they continue to do what is wrong?

Taking this treasure to heart. **What is one nugget of truth God is teaching you today?**

Review Briefly: Protein, Omega 3, Fish and Eggs (pp. 149-154) if time permits.

Explain: **In Luke 11 you read about Jesus comparing two foods. In each one there is a clean food and an unclean food. Jesus refers to these clean foods as good gifts.**

Read: Matthew 5:17.

Did Jesus come to abolish the law? What does that tell us about the law in regards to your answer? (p. 156)

No, the laws are still for our health today as they were when they were written.

Explain: **Three excuses people use to eat what they want. (pp. 155-157)**

1. *Cooking temperature. Do you feel that this would make a difference between clean and unclean?*
2. *Peter's vision. Does this make all foods clean?*
3. *Giving thanks erases the uncleanness. Does this make sense?*

Review First 6 weeks: (If time permits this is a good exercise to show the value of their learning and all we have covered in our treasure adventure.)

Let's review the treasure chest: This four step visual process reminds participants of the health problems they once were dealing with and how God's foods can heal.

Step 1 - What foods did you once eat?

Using a black marker, write on a dry-erase board the foods mentioned such as pop tarts, chips, cookies, hamburger helper, mac and cheese – Kraft, etc. List all the foods in large letters so the words cover the entire board. The words can be written in different angles, crowded and overlapping. The idea is to show a collage of words representing the food choices we made.

Step 2 - Now write out the symptoms we were dealing with as a result from these foods.

Overwrite the foods written on the board with a different colored marker such as red. When you finish this step the board should look like a mess but with the words still distinguishable. Answers might include: allergies, asthma, cancer, diabetes, lethargy, etc...

Step 3 - Now what foods have we studied that will give us health and that can replace the other foods we were eating?

For this step give each person a piece of colored construction paper in a size that is appropriate for the single word to be written on it. Then have them write the food name on it. I.e. one piece of paper might say banana, another might have written zucchini, or fresh milled bread, or tomato, etc. If you have a small group then give each person enough pieces of paper for the board to be filled when completed. The idea of this step is to show with an assortment of colors the goodness God has given us in place of the foods we were once choosing. Have each person tape the construction paper on the board covering up the previous illness words.

Step 4 – What scripture verses have been your guide so far on this journey?

Ask 4 or 5 people to write out a significant verse they discovered on this treasure hunt. Write either the scripture reference or the entire scripture on construction paper. Tape these to the board at the bottom and sides of the collection of food papers to show a foundation and border. The result should be a very colorful arrangement of words signifying the bounty of foods gifted to us and found in God's Word. With all of these treasures come the blessings of health, vitality, freedom from illness, energy, fellowship, insight and blessings

Now that we have fully learned the value of God's treasure, it is up to us to protect this treasure chest. We must be on guard from the Trojan horses in our culture. Many things can slip in and distract us from our goal and gradually take our eyes off the treasure. Then we will begin to look again to man's plans. Just as we are cautioned to hide God's Word in our heart, we need to guard against any imitations threatening to snatch away what we have learned.

Don't miss Part II when the hidden pirates are unveiled that want to threaten the treasure. As you protect the treasure you will learn even more ways to enhance the bounty so that it will benefit your family and those around you even more.

TASTE AND SEE

Grocery Tips: Meat – check date on package, buy the latest date. If the package is drippy and sticky – avoid! If fish smells fishy – avoid. Color is not an indicator of value in meat, since most of it is added, but if the coloring looks off to you then it is not a good purchase. Meat should not have an odor – if it does, don't eat it. The best choice is organic or from a farmer you have met and talked with to see if the animals were allowed to roam in the fields eating grass and are not antibiotic treated.

VIDEO: Dr. Couey: Controlling Inflammation and the Couey 6-Week Challenge
This video covers the material in the *Nutrition Manual* pages 219-225. It is helpful to have the book open for reference during the talk.

◆ ◆ ◆

VIEWER GUIDE ANSWERS

God made our body out of 27 chemicals.

100,000 chemical reactions per second.

There are approximately 20,000 enzymes in the human body.
1. Nutrition - cells getting the proper amount of the 27 chemicals.
2. Oxygen – to create energy we must exercise
3. Waste Removal
   a) Limit saturated fat
   b) Exercise
   c) Hydrate
   Spiritual attitudes also affect your body chemistry.

Protein membranes:
- Open with positive self-talk
- Negativity causes it to shut down
- Opens widest with laughter
- Opens when we are happy, kind and giving
- Avoid anger, fear and depression
- Prayers opens the protein membrane

◆ ◆ ◆

WRAP IT UP

Dr. Couey mentioned the pH of water. A pH test kit can be purchased at pet stores used for aquariums or at pool supply stores. He also mentioned glycemic index of foods. This can be found in numerous internet locations and there is no one list better than others. They are all stating the facts.

HOMEWORK

Read Part II and Fasting/ Self-Discipline.

Try one new recipe this week. Begin going back to old recipes, family favorites, exchanging the ingredients for healthier choices. Bring in these transformed recipes along with samples for everyone to try.

VIDEO: Conclusion of Part I

CLOSE IN PRAYER.

PART II

Week Seven

Fasting — Steps to Self-Control

AGENDA

Welcome

Prayer and Praise Tickles

Discussion: Part II Focus*

    The content of this lesson may require diligence in time monitoring.

Video: Fasting Intro (2 minutes)

    Review: Fasting (25 minutes)

    Daniel Fast (20 minutes)

    Taste and See (15 minutes)

    Video: Steps to Self- Control (45 minutes)

    Wrap It Up

BRING

- Suggested foods: Black Bean Soup or Butternut Squash Soup

DVD 4

- Printed copy of the Daniel Fast booklet found on the website under books. It is also available on Kindle.

> These notes on fasting are lengthy and your class time may not permit reviewing in full detail. A suggested approach would be to study this leader guide before class time and then highlight the questions you wish to review.

WELCOME

PRAYER and PRAISE TICKLES

DISCUSSION: In the first half of this journey we focused on how to build our health bank account. We've talked about the value of our treasure chest and the bounty it contains. Now we move on to the protection phase.

Protection of our treasure will be an on-going battle against the pirates. These pirates come in the form of wrong information, health matters that do not follow the three principles, and information void God's Word. It is necessary to thoroughly review all information to determine if it follows biblical guidelines.

Health is important. It helps us reach our potential for God's will. It is not an end in and of itself. It is a benefit of following God's commands. In today's society more and more people are focused on food. We have an opportunity to show them God's food book and how applying this book to their health will enable them to apply it to their whole life. Do we want healthy relationships? Do we want to understand money? Do we want confidence? Are we content in the situation we are in? Our study is showing us that we must look to God as our Provider for health and life. We can then transfer this knowledge to all areas of our lives. In order to do so, we must constantly be on guard to protect our treasure and add to it.

Our first stop in Part II of this study is to understand God's Word regarding fasting and self- discipline. We will spend a lot of time reviewing this chapter because it is pivotal in a Christian's walk with the Lord. If this subject is new to you, please consider how God might use this in your life. If you will continue to ask Him, he will reveal to you, in His time, how He wants you to apply this knowledge. Because it's new, it might be easy to "skip over" this section thinking it doesn't apply to you. Please keep asking him. If you choose to ignore this area, you may very well miss out on what could be a major blessing in your Christian walk.

Share Rhonda Sutton's testimony from the Daniel Fast booklet, printed from the website.

VIDEO: Fasting Intro

REVIEW: Fasting (pages 169-183)

Fasting is defined as abstaining from food, either completely or partially, for a specified period of time. It refers to self-denial.

This subject has been neglected in our churches and in our spheres of influence.
> **Because of this lack of knowledge what concerns did you write down in regards to fasting?**
> **Would anyone like to share your concerns? (p. 170)**

In your lesson you were asked to look up Isaiah 58:1-6. Verse 6 points out ways fasting will help us. What are they? (p. 171)
> *Lose the bonds of wickedness to undo the heavy burdens, to set the oppressed free, and break every yoke.*

John Piper, a well-known author and pastor, gives us his insight into fasting: (*It might be helpful to write these points on the board before class starts in case the class wants a copy.*)
1) Fasting has a long and righteous history with Christians.
2) Fasting can reveal things that are in our hearts and that control us.
3) Fasting is an important spiritual discipline that draws us closer to God and glorifies Him.

4) Fasting (along with prayer) is one of the most effective ways of showing God our "hunger" for Him.

5) Fasting for the right reasons will bring us immeasurable gifts from our Father.
   Wrong reason – to bring glory to ourselves

   Piper goes on to explain that understanding the teachings of Isaiah 58 holds the key to fasting for the glory of God. We fast as an offering of emptiness to God in hope. It signifies our utter helplessness and total dependence on God.

Our goal for fasting, as with any discipline in our Christian walk, is freedom. If the result is not greater freedom, then something is wrong. There will be times in your life when fasting is necessary to break the bonds of strongholds such as gossiping, alcohol, food addictions, lack of trust, sinful behaviors and so on. Turning your problems over to God and letting Him take control over these areas will bring this freedom and a great yoke will be lifted from your shoulders. Discipline always has its rewards.

John Piper also states:

Our "duty" as Christians is to delight ourselves in intimacy with our Heavenly Father. He speaks of the power of prayer and fasting and how these disciplines -- which seem to be so tedious, so difficult, so "duty like" -- actually release some of the greatest freedom and gives us the greatest joy we can experience in this life.

In your lesson you looked up several verses regarding individuals who fasted for various situations. (pp. 172-173)

Who were some of those people you read about in Scripture?

Were any of these fasting references new to you?

Own answers

From this reading what is one truth you learned in regards to fasting?

Own answers

SPIRITUAL BENEFITS OF FASTING (p.174)

Of the 20 benefits listed on pages 174-175, which one caught your attention the most?

Sometimes when God calls you to fast, it may be for only one of these reasons. There may be other times that He calls you to practice fasting for many or all of these reasons. Keep track of these reasons on the Fasting Track Sheet found in the *Nutrition Manual* (p. 266).

The Billy Graham web site states:

"Fasting can be a wonderful spiritual experience. Believers who never practice fasting and prayer are missing a spiritual discipline that has blessed many throughout the ages." Can you give an accurate citation for this?

Fasting is not only for our benefit but can be done by us for the benefit of others. Is there someone in your life who desperately needs God to work in their life? Is God calling you to intercede for them by fasting and praying specifically for this person and this issue? (p. 175)

It has been reported Shirley Dobson fasted one day a week to fervently pray for her husband and kids. Though our families may not be in the public eye such as Dr. James Dobson (founder of Focus on the Family), it is no less important to pray for them fervently and sacrificially.

What questions do you have in regards to the spiritual benefits of fasting?

PHYSICAL BENEFITS OF FASTING (P. 176)

A person in good health may choose not to eat occasional meals in order to focus on devotion to God. Not only are there spiritual benefits, but some doctors believe that there are also health benefits. The early church found prayer and fasting valuable when seeking the guidance of the Holy Spirit for making important decisions such as choosing spiritual leaders. (see Acts 13:2-3 and 14:23) God will honor and bless anyone who fasts and prays in the right spirit.

Additional physical benefits of fasting:
Promotes healing, lowers cholesterol, lowers blood pressure, relieves arthritis, stops loss of bone mass, relieves joint pain, relieves morning stiffness, has calming effect, increases mental alertness, stops food addictions

Share: Stories from Dr. Rex Russell.
1) Sue, a bright, cute nine-year old, had severe dyslexia. Her loving and interested family had the financial resources to take her to the best medical facilities in the country for evaluation. She was being tutored by a teacher who was an expert in learning problems. At one point, Sue became ill with the flu and couldn't eat for several days. When the teacher returned, he found to his surprise that Sue could read! He remarked to the parents, "I don't know what you are doing but please don't quit. She is reading above her expected reading level."

Does this mean that rest, fever and fasting will correct dyslexia? No.

When Sue resumed her normal diet, her reading problems returned. Later, when she experimented and ate only unfamiliar foods, her reading skill improved. Further testing revealed that she was sensitive to sugar, corn, white flour, margarine, honey and several other frequently eaten foods. As you might suspect, the foods she liked best were the most offending.

2) Another observation occurred in Dr. Russell's immediate family. They had a son who was hyperactive. Several kinds of therapy proved unsatisfactory. Another plan included a three-day fast prior to treatment. Having never considered fasting before, the Russell's were a little scared and apprehensive. Rather than water fast, (What does this mean?) they let their son eat only foods he had never eaten before—plums, kiwis, fish, and cashews and so on. They were absolutely astounded by the third day to see him being calm. They thought he was lethargic, but

he was probably just acting normal. Many of his favorite foods stimulated him to the extremes of activity and a lack of concentration. Of course, it was hard—almost impossible—to keep him interested in eating certain foods instead of junk foods, so their troubles had not completely ended. They decided to investigate further into what happens when the body is deprived of certain foods. They looked into fasting.

TYPES OF FASTING (P. 177)

What are the three types of fasting? (write this on the board so everyone can see it.)

1. Normal - no food, but water

2. Absolute - no food or water

3. Partial – omitting one meal a day or certain foods for a specific time period; i.e. just drinking vegetable or fruit juices

   (Some authors also list a 4th type called Rotational. A rotational fast omits certain foods for a period of time, primarily for the purpose of determining allergies.)

SLEEP, REST AND FASTING

These teaching notes are helpful to understand how fasting is beneficial for illness but if time is limited they are easy to skip over.

What is one of the main benefits of a good night's sleep?

A chance for the body to heal and rest, particularly the digestive system

From the very beginning, before the Fall of humans, our bodies were designed to take periodic rests from food. The seventh day was designed for rest, and the digestive system needs rest just as much as our physical body does. When we sleep at night our digestive system gets a rest. This allows it to catch up and let the immune system do its job. Have you ever started the morning off with a lot of congestion? This is the stuff your body has been busy trying to clean out of your system while you slept. And if you take an antihistamine to dry it up then it will have to work again to try and get rid of it another way. Instead, let your body heal itself and if a symptom continues, you may be able to heal naturally by changing your diet or by using supplements.

What are the three ways your body was designed to respond to sickness?

Fever, fasting, rest

Your body was designed to respond to sickness with a fever. When we have a fever, we crave rest, not food. Do you remember the last time you were sick? Did you want to eat? Did you want to party? No. You had a temperature, could not keep any food down and only wanted to crawl into your bed and be left alone.

Why do we work so hard to lower our temperatures? Fever causes us to ache and to want to lie down. We fight to "keep going" because of the many pressures of our daily lives. We don't want to appear weak or let someone down. Fever, rest and fasting are a part of the design to shorten viral infections.

Briefly review: In week #1 we learned that health begins at the cellular level.

Healthy (cells) make healthy (tissues) which make healthy (organs) which make a healthy organ (system). How can we apply fasting to the health of our cells?

If we want to be healthy we need to begin by giving our cells times to rest. A good night's sleep gives our body the ability to repair itself much more quickly. If you get some real rest as soon as you have a viral infection, it will likely last fewer days than the average. Also, in Week 6 we learned that garlic, onions, alfalfa, and vitamin C will greatly speed up recovery time.

Why do we tend not to fast?

We enjoy eating. We don't understand fasting.

***DANIEL FAST – This part of the study will be very instrumental to each participant when applied. Take time in class to review each question in the book and compare answers to your discoveries. Ask each participant to be prayerful in regards to fasting. Take time now to pray about this discipline and how each individual will be able to implement it into their diet for the next 21 days.

An email list could be gathered for those who want to fast and write encouragement emails to each other during the 21 day fast.

Commitment cards are found on the last page of the Daniel Fast booklet. These can be copied for each participant to sign one copy for the leader (or Daniel Fast leader) and keep the other one for them.

Ask those in classes who wish to not participate to pray for those who do. If a person is not capable of participating in the fast at this time ask them to fast from something in their lifestyle – like watching TV or some other time consuming activity and then use this time saved for devotion to God.

Review pages 182-183 with the class and ask them for their answers to the questions.

Daniel made up his mind to follow through.

There is a Daniel Fast booklet on the Designed Healthy Living website that gives instructions, menus and recipes.

Everyone can do a fast – they just need to determine what type will fit their health program.

Making this commitment and then helping them follow through will be a major breakthrough in their Christian walk. Be an encourager.

Families and the Daniel Fast – Implementing this fast is great for families to do together. Read aloud the story of Daniel to your kids and then have the kids act out the different scenes. Follow through with eating Daniel's power foods. Ask your kids if they want to be smarter or faster in three weeks then they are today? Have fun doing timed races or other events to record times. Then after following this fast – re-record the times. The families that have made this a fun learning experience did not have any trouble getting the family members on board with this fast. Those who made it a list of rules had a revolt.

TASTE AND SEE

Here are some foodie notes to share with the group if time permits.

FOODIE NOTES:

Encourage them to make these immediate easy changes:

1. Switch from white refined rice to brown rice. If you need a transition step for your family, try Uncle Ben's Converted Rice or wild rice. Your ultimate goal is to resort to the brown rice.

2. Change from refined flour pasta to whole wheat, spelt, or rice pasta, or better yet – freshly milled flour.

3. From microwave popcorn, change to organic popcorn made the old fashioned way on the stove or in a hot air popcorn maker. Use seasoning salt that doesn't have MSG. Cook in butter or olive oil.

4. Look for whole grain cereals with a honey or fruit juice sweetener. Kashi is a brand that is usually whole grain. Read the labels. The label will indicate if it uses whole grain.

5. If you like grits, you can make your own with a Vita Mix rather than using the refined grits in the box that aren't fresh.

♦ ♦ ♦

VIDEO: Four Steps to Self-Control

There are no fill-in blanks for this session. This video will cover the problem with addictions, more specifically food addictions although the truths presented can be applied to all addictive behaviors. There is a second hand-out titled Overcoming Compulsive Overeating. This title will not attract many people to pick it up but it does apply to numerous people thin and overweight. It is helpful to go ahead and print out one copy for everyone instead of having participants pick one up from a table. This is a "closet" problem that is rarely admitted.

There is an eating disorder epidemic in America and of the people plagued not everyone shows it in their dress size. Even thin people can have an eating disorder.

♦ ♦ ♦

WRAP IT UP

HOMEWORK

Read Week 8, "Sweets," in the Bible study, and pages 103-121 in the *Nutrition Manual*. Look for various kinds of sweeteners and bring them to class next week.

Try a favorite recipe and replace the sweetener with honey.

Next Week's Topic Teaser: *Sweets are the most desired foods but how do they affect our immune system?*

CLOSE IN PRAYER.

Week Eight
Sweets—Solutions for Our Immune System

AGENDA

    Welcome

    Prayer and Praise Tickles

    Review: previous weeks (10 minutes)

    Video: Sweets Intro (1:30 minutes)

    Review: Sweets (40 minutes)

    Taste and See (10 minutes)

    Video: Solutions for Our Immune System (45 minutes) (Ellie Cullen, RN)

    Wrap It Up

BRING

- Look for cookbooks that incorporate honey instead of sugar. These are becoming more common place.
- Bring in an assortment of sweeteners such as brown rice syrup, agave, Sweet Leaf, molasses, raw honey, honey in the rough, honey comb, etc. It is fun to try each one on a toothpick to savor the difference.
- Suggested Foods: Surprise Brownies and Healthy Banana Cookies
- DVD 5
- See page 53 for class demo ideas.

WELCOME

PRAYER AND PRAISE TICKLES

REVIEW: Weeks 1-7:

    What did we learn about water?

    What beverages are best to drink?

    What beverages should be limited or eliminated?

    What did we learn about grains?

    How do we apply the three principles to grains?

    How can we apply what we learned to our celebrations?

    What did we learn about fruits and vegetables?

What quality nutrients can be obtained from these foods?

How do we apply the three principles to these foods?

What did we learn about oil, herbs and spices?

How can you enhance your holiday menus with these?

What did we learn about meats?

In Leviticus what meats are good for us to eat?

From what we know in today's science, why is that true?

How do we apply the three principles to meat?

Of all the foods we studied, which ones have the most antioxidants?

What foods can contribute to the most free radicals?

If you were to look at the treasure chest filled only with foods God has given us, what would you see? Do you want to protect it?

How will fasting protect our treasure?

What is a benefit of self-discipline?

VIDEO: Sweets Intro

REVIEW: Sweets

In the house of the wise are stores of choice food and oil. (Proverbs 21:20)
Sweets are definitely the choice food for many people.

Let's review the three principles? Ask a different person to quote this each time.
1. *Eat only substances God created for food.*
2. *As much as possible, eat foods as they were created.*
3. *Avoid food addictions.*

Now let's apply them to sugar:
1. *Eat sugars in the items God created as food.*

What would be an example? fruit
2. *Eat sugars before they are changed into what man thinks is better.*

What is an example of something that has been changed? refined sugar
3. *Don't be addicted to sugar.*

What is an example of something sweet we can be addicted to? chocolate, desserts
> *God gave us a taste pallet, a specific place on our tongue that allows us to enjoy sweets. We've been taking advantage of that.*

Share: *Around the time of the American Revolution, the average American consumed approximately 5 pounds of sugar per year. Today, the average American is consuming anywhere from 147 - 160 pounds per year! Tests have shown that* *when we consume 24 teaspoons of sugar in one day, our immune system is depressed by 92%. The average is 42 teaspoons a day. Approximately 30 percent of the US dollar is spent on food containing sugar.*

What are we doing to our immune system? We get mad at God for the breakdown of our bodies. What if the real reason is that we are consuming too much sugar? Try to cut back on your refined sugar and sugar substitutes. Always read the ingredients of products you buy. One teaspoon of sugar equals 4 grams.

What a difference it would make in attitudes, health, emotions, attention, etc. in our children if they didn't buy treats from the vending machine. Be aware of the facts.

CLASS DEMONSTRATION:

Show calculations of sugar grams of a typical daily diet. You can do this by bringing in packages of food from your pantry and then calculating the sugar grams. A bag of organic granola lists 9 grams of sugar for each ½ cup serving. This would mean it has over 2 teaspoons of sugar per serving. This particular granola is low in sugar compared to most packaged foods. Raisins have 29 gms. sugar for each ¼ cup.

Bring in food samples or packages to calculate sugar grams. A healthy cereal such as Cascadian Farms is organic but still includes a lot of sugar.

Tips for this demo: Plan out a full day of typical foods. Here are some ideas. Write these out on the marker board:

Breakfast: Sweetened vanilla almond milk, Cascadian farms organic cereal. = 30 gms 7 teaspoons sugar

Lunch: salad, fruit, dressing, sweetened green tea = 10-20 gms. 2 ½ - 5 teaspoons sugar

Snack: French vanilla yogurt, 0% fat 22 grams sugar with granola = 31 gms. = 10 teaspoons sugar

Dinner: Vegetable Stir Fry – 7 gms sugar, apple cranberry quinoa – 4 gms sugar, applesauce (homemade) 3 gms. sugar, dinner roll = 14 + gms. sugar = 4 teaspoons sugar

This day's menu seems fairly healthy but yet the sugar is still a total of 26 teaspoons sugar. The National average is 30-50 teaspoons per day.

Point of this demo: Natural foods contain fructose, a more desirable sugar for the body and specifically the pancreas. Be aware of how much sugar is in processed foods, including healthy choices. Make alternative choices that would reduce the total amount of sugar.

> Foodie Facts: One candy bar = the sugar in 10 apples!
>
> 4 grams of sugar = 1 teaspoon
>
> Eating processed sugar diminishes your immune system for 4 hours.

Honey (pages 195-199)

What sweetener did God give us and how many times is it mentioned in Scripture?

Honey – 40 times

What did we learn from Proverbs 24:13?

Honey includes many important vitamins and minerals such as 18 amino acids, protein, enzymes, fats, vitamins, minerals, elements, trace elements, good acids, etc… The point is that God gave us a sweetener with nutritional value. There are over 165 ingredients in honey that God has placed there to work for our good. Enzymes break down the sugar for our body to use. Refined sugar doesn't do this. Honey is absorbed more slowly than sugar.

Is all honey the same?

No

What should we shop for?

Raw, unpasteurized honey.

Heat honey only with other ingredients to prevent loss of its benefits, such as in the fresh milled bread. There are many types of honey. Mild includes tupelo, sage, clover. Strong includes sour wood and buckwheat. Diabetics should use sage or tupelo because it contains levulose. Levulose helps keep blood sugar more stable.

Why buy honey locally?

Builds immunity to many allergies.

What is interesting about chemical sprays that may be present on the plants from which the bees collect honey?

The chemicals are not transferred to the honey.

Honey is another beautiful design by our Creator who cares for us. God has done everything to give us His divine provisions.

Share: <u>One pound</u> of honey contains:

1.4 gm. protein	23 mg calcium	73 mg phosphorus	4.1 mg iron
0.02 riboflavin	1.0 niacin	16 mg vitamin C	360.0 carbs
1,333 calories			

HONEY FACTS

- Honey is the best sweetener for the kidneys to process because it is free of bacteria.
- One tablespoon of honey is equal in sweetness to 5 tablespoons of sugar.

The Problems of Sugar (pp. 202-208)

Explain: Simple sugars require B-Complex to be digested and metabolized. All natural carbohydrates have an abundance of B-Complex so the body can assimilate them well.

What happens when manufacturers remove the B vitamins?

Our body must supply them from other areas.

A depletion of B vitamins results in what?

Mood swings, heart problems, etc.

If you must eat sugar, make sure you eat plenty of fiber along with it. Remember, we get B vitamins from whole grains.

Discuss: Aspartame, Splenda, and artificial sweeteners (pages 206-207) if time permits.

TASTE and SEE

Enjoy the foods your class members have prepared.

♦ ♦ ♦

VIDEO: Solutions for Our Immune System, (Ellie Cullen, RN, Founder: Your Future Health, www.yourfuture-health.com)

VIEWER GUIDE TO ANSWERS

Sugar and the Immune System

The immune system protects the body from foreign substances like heavy metals such as <u>mercury,</u> <u>lead</u> and <u>arsenic.</u> And pathogenic organisms like bacteria, viruses and parasites.

Overload leads to <u>disease.</u>

GLUTATHIONE acts as a major <u>detoxifier.</u>

<u>Stress</u> can severely reduce or kill the very nutrients needed to make glutathione.

<u>Stress</u> is the number one enemy of the immune system.

A, B, C, D, E, and the minerals <u>zinc</u> and <u>iron.</u>

The thyroid cleans the blood every <u>17</u> minutes.

One food that will undermine all these efforts - <u>sugar</u>

Sugar is the number one enemy of the <u>pancreas.</u>

◆ ◆ ◆

WRAP IT UP

HOMEWORK

Read more about the immune system on pages 211-225 in the *Nutrition Manual.*

Read Week Nine in the Bible study.

CLOSE IN PRAYER.

Week Nine

Environment & Toxins — PROTECTION: Increasing Our Value

AGENDA

    Welcome

    Prayer and Praise Tickles

    Review: previous weeks (10 minutes)

    Video: Toxins Intro (2 minutes)

    Review: Environment & Toxins (30 minutes)

    Taste and See (10 minutes)

    Video: Protection: Increasing Our Personal Value (45 minutes)

    *Video Follow Up: **Highly Recommended**! (20 minutes)

    Wrap It Up

BRING

- Suggested Foods: Roasted Sweet Potatoes and Scalloped Turnips.
- DVD 6
- Basic H2 sample from Full Study Kit – made into a window cleaner and an all- purpose cleaner.
- The video session this week is going to list several resources such as Shaklee and foamer bottles. It would be helpful to have samples on hand or a sign-up sheet for those who might want you to place a group order. Shaklee can be purchased through distributors. Contact the Designed Healthy Living office or website to locate a distributor in your area. The foamer bottles can be purchased through various websites, but the most economical is bottlesandfoamers.com.

(Shaklee does have a membership available for those who are interested. If that is not preferred and your group just wants to get the Basic H2 bottles that will last up to 3 years, then contact the Designed Healthy Living office to place an order at member price without setting up a membership.)

It is imperative that you preview **before class** the second video and the viewer guide, "Protection: Increasing Our Personal Value." How thoroughly you are prepared beforehand will greatly impact the effectiveness of the message, since it does not have a corresponding book assignment. You will need extra time **in** class for each participant to write out their Proverbs 31 affirmations and reveal them to the group. The value of saying these affirmations out loud is priceless. God's Words spoken in personal form really reaches down into each person's heart. Continue to be prayerful for your class. Many people are hurting and this class can help them release that hurt.

The toxins in the home can be previewed before class by studying Healthy Home in the Nutrition Manual, pages 217-241. This will help you be fully prepared for class and any questions that may arise.

WELCOME

PRAYER AND PRAISE TICKLES

What have you seen God doing around you that you may have missed before taking this class?

What health reports do you have about how changing foods already has made a difference?

REVIEW: previous weeks

How has your view of foods changed?

How has your view of your body changed?

How has your view of your relationship with God changed?

Last week we looked at how sugar can deplete our immune system and our health. How did you handle sugar this past week?

VIDEO: Toxins Intro

REVIEW: Environment and Toxins

This week you read about the environment and toxins. The reading assignment was lengthy with less interactive work. I hope you were able to glean some valuable truths about toxins.

Day 1: Removing Decay from the Treasure (p. 217)

What did you learn about Jehoshaphat?

He became king, the Lord was with him, and he did not seek idols

What is Jehoshaphat's recommendation in response to King Ahab's desire to invade a neighboring country?

Inquire of the Lord first

What was Jehoshaphat's first reaction and his response when he heard that Judah was about to be invaded?

Afraid, turned his attention to seek the Lord, proclaimed a fast.

Then he stood before the people and gave a mighty prayer.

Look at page 218 in your books.

Have someone read the "fill in the blanks" section for 2 Chronicles 20?

Verse 9: *we will stand before this house… thy name is in this house*

Verse 12: *Our eyes are on Thee*

Verse 15: *Do not fear or be dismayed*

Verse 17: *Do not fear or be dismayed for the Lord is with you*

In these verses we read that the battle is not ours but God's.

Still on page 218, would someone read verse 20?

Another person read verse 21?

Later in our lesson today we are going to revisit these verses.

For now, how can we apply Jehoshaphat's situation to our situation?

We too need to stand before our houses and protect them.

PRAY

This is a good time to have prayer. Pray for the people in the class not to be afraid, because the Lord is with them.

Which part of the body is the Toxin Terminator?

The liver

What did you learn about the liver?

The liver is responsible for detoxification, metabolism, and storage of nutrients.

Would you want to be without any of these functions in your body?

No

How can we assist the liver in its duties?

Eat foods from the Mediterranean pyramid – lots of fruits and veggies – raw

How are we getting contaminants in our body?

Food and food containers, tap water, skin care products, air pollution, and cleaners we use on our clothes and dishes.

In the lesson under DAY 2 look at the list of symptoms on page 223, how did your list look when you finished?

Were you surprised by this?

Are you ready to get rid of these invaders?

This is an area where you are in charge to a large degree. We control what gets brought into our homes, what we eat, and what we put on our skin. Be encouraged. Realize this is an amazing step forward toward great health improvements.

Did you take inventory of your home cleaners? (pp. 224-225)

Did you find many problems lurking in your home?

Your study gave you a list of 7 things you can do to clean your home and protect your health at the same time. (pp. 226-227)

Which of these are you willing to do?

Then in Day 3 of the study; What did you learn about the personal care products you are using?

What is the acid mantle?

God designed our skin to have an acid mantle. It is a very fine, slightly acidic film on the surface acting as a barrier to bacteria, viruses and other potential contaminants that may penetrate the skin. Antibacterial cleaners remove this acid mantle and our protection.

Do you have any pH balanced products in your home?

Then on Day 4 of this study it talked about allergies; how can we apply these principles to allergies?

1. *Eating foods designed by God rarely leads to allergies.*
2. *Eating foods as close as possible to God's design will help us avoid most allergies. These foods will keep our digestive tract healthy which will decrease the chances of leaky gut and other problems*
3. *Addictions are a sign there is an allergy of some sort. Recognizing this will tell us we have a problem that needs correcting.*

The bottom line is: now you have the information you need to make healthy choices and reverse many symptoms. **What are you going to do with this knowledge?**

TASTE and SEE

Enjoy the foods the class has prepared.

♦ ♦ ♦

VIDEO: Protection: Increasing Our Personal Value

This lesson will require more time.   See note in the Agenda.

VIEWER GUIDE TO ANSWERS

<u>All</u> that a man achieves or fails to achieve is a direct result of his <u>self-talk.</u> – John Maxwell

Established means – <u>Thrive</u> or grow <u>successfully</u>

Our self-talk affects our <u>destiny</u>.

Our state of mind affects the health of our <u>cells</u>.

VIDEO FOLLOW UP - See notes in the beginning of today's lesson.

♦ ♦ ♦

WRAP IT UP

HOMEWORK

Read Week 10, "Stress and Forgiveness," in *Treasures*.
Read pages 251-259 in the *Nutrition Manual*.

NEXT WEEK'S TOPIC TEASER: *Next week we will hear some powerful testimonies on forgiveness.*

CLOSE IN PRAYER.

Week Ten
Stress & Forgiveness — From Bitterness to Freedom

AGENDA

> Welcome
>
> Prayer and Praise Tickles
>
> Video: No video intro this week.
>
> Review: Stress & Forgiveness (30 minutes)
>
> Taste and See (10 minutes)
>
> Video: From Bitterness to Freedom (50 minutes)
>
> Wrap It Up

BRING

- Suggested foods include Marinated Vegetable Salad and Spicy Warm Black Bean Dip.
- DVD 5

PREPARATION: Note the video is 65 minutes so plan class accordingly. The testimonies presented are powerful. A box of tissues may be needed. Be prepared with contact information of a pastor or counselor either written on the board or as a handout.

WELCOME

PRAYER and PRAISE TICKLES

REVIEW: Stress & Forgiveness

Can someone please read Isaiah 40:29-31?
Encourage students to memorize these verses.

Who do you think this verse is referring to when it says "the weary"?
fatigued, tired, exhausted, worn out, drained

Do you lack might (strength, power, capacity)?

Are you weary? What promise does He give us (the weary)?

We will gain new strength, will fly like eagles, will run and not get tired will walk and not get weary.

When you are stressed are you weary and/or do you lack might?

Eagles are mentioned throughout Scripture and each time they are viewed as a magnificent bird with great power, strength, speed, and awesome wonder. Their wings spread out 90 inches.

The poem (on page 244) by Stacy Smith is for you to read when times are tough. When we can rise above our circumstances and see from an eagle's viewpoint, we can escape from the impending trouble and see things from God's perspective. Two important points are to step away from a situation (even if only mentally) and then view it from God's perspective. This is the beginning of release from stress.

What does James 1:2 tell us?

Have someone read this from their homework.

Is stress good or bad?

Can be both.

How would you describe stress after studying your lesson?

Own answers.

What are the four main causes of stress?

Environment, diet, exercise, attitude

Looking at this list – how many of these are you unable to control?

With God's guidance we are able to control all areas but it may seem like we cannot at times.

Review the listed causes of stress you are experiencing. What areas need attention?

Symptoms of stress (pages 246-248) & (*Nutrition Manual* pages 253 – 259)

Review these symptoms and help participants find applicable solutions for stress.

Now that we have learned how our body responds, let's look back at our study:

In Jonah 2:2, what did Jonah do in this time of stress?

Cried out to God.

Can we do this also?

YES

Which of the verses on pages 250-252 stood out to you in regards to stress?

Which ones would be good to memorize or have written down for future stress?

Review 1 Peter 5:7. How did this verse speak to you?

Would anyone like to share the affirmation they wrote? (p. 252)

From pages 253-257How did you finish the statement: You know you are stressed when you _____?

Read Mark 6:31. What does "a lonely place" mean?

Own answers.

Can you think of a place where you can go?

In the margin of your study guide write down that place and then beside it write down a time when you want to plan to go there.

Read Isaiah 41:10, 13.

From page 258, have someone read each one of these verses and then comment on its significance to forgiveness.

Psalm 103:5

Who satisfies your years with good things, so that your youth is renewed like the eagles?

Isaiah 40:31

Yet those that wait for the Lord will gain new strength; they will mount up with wings like eagles, they will run and not get tired, they will walk and not become weary.

Exodus 19:4

You yourselves have seen what I did to the Egyptians, and how I bore you on eagle's wings and brought you to Myself.

TASTE and SEE

Enjoy the good food the class members have brought in.

◆ ◆ ◆

VIDEO: See notes at beginning of lesson.

Right now, before the video begins, pray and fully believe that "God has a great work here to be done" in your life. God LOVES you and has prepared this time, and these testimonies from Jane Elder and Sue Becker, to "continue the good work He has begun in you" (Philippians 1:6)

First testimony is Jane Elder, notes of her talk are on the handout. There are no fill-ins so people can focus on what is being said.

This is followed by Sue Becker's testimony.

VIEWER GUIDE ANSWERS for Sue Becker's testimony:

The Healing Power of Forgiveness

She asked God, "have I ever heard from you --- what is this all about?" But even in the middle of her question, she says that "God remained <u>faithful</u>.

Jeremiah 17 says "the heart is <u>deceitful</u> above all things, who can know it".

We deceive ourselves because we <u>justify</u> things.

Doctors can deal with that tumor but only God can deal with your <u>heart.</u>

2 Chronicle 7:14 *If My people, who are called by My name, will <u>humble</u> themselves and pray, and turn from their wicked ways, then I will hear from heaven and heal their land.*

Recognize unforgiveness as your <u>own sin.</u>

As surely as you are <u>physical</u> you are spiritual

As surely as you are <u>spiritual</u> you are physical.

◆ ◆ ◆

WRAP IT UP

HOMEWORK

Read Week 11 "Exercise and Scripture Memory."

Read page 245 in the *Nutrition Manual.*

Start sign-ups for the final week's banquet. If you are inviting guests to the banquet such as spouse or church staff begin a sign-up sheet for this also so that you can be prepared with seating.

CLOSE IN PRAYER.

Week Eleven

Exercise and Scripture Memory — Made to Move

AGENDA

Welcome

Prayer and Praise Tickles

Review: previous weeks (15 minutes)

Video: Exercise Intro (3 minutes)

Video: Body & Soul – Optional (4 minutes)

Review: Exercise and Scripture Memory

Taste and See (10 minutes)

Video: Made to Move (37 minutes)

Wrap-Up

BRING

- Suggested foods: Kids Energy Bars and Dried Fruit Balls
- Bring sign-up sheet for final week banquet.
- DVD 6

WELCOME

PRAYER and PRAISE TICKLES

Action Plan: Time to check in and see how everyone is doing at making one simple plan per week to implement the teachings of this study.

REVIEW: previous weeks – use own notes

VIDEO: Exercise Intro

VIDEO: Body & Soul – this is a Christian fitness program that your church or group may be interested in. Class time may not allow viewing it but it would be good to show as people are arriving or leaving.

REVIEW: Exercise and Scripture Memory

Most of us have set various goals for exercise and some of us have experienced success but many of us suffer from a failure to follow through.

Someone please read Psalm 139:14. Is this verse a motivator?

Note the list of reasons why exercise is important on page 270.

Share: 40% of people get cancer; however of those who exercise, only 14% get cancer.

Someone please read I Corinthians 6:19-20. Why is it important to protect and preserve our temple?

Occupancy by the Holy Spirit, Ownership by the Lord, Obedience to the Lord

Ask students to share their ideas for motivation to exercise on page 273.

I Corinthians 9:24-27 tells us: "So run that you may obtain it [the prize]; Every athlete exercises self-control in all things...I discipline my body and keep it under control, lest after preaching to others I myself should be disqualified."

Our God requires us to practice self-control in all aspects of life. We do this not only in obedience, but also to display to the world the difference that Christ makes in us. Exercise is a discipline: other training that develops and molds who we are physically, mentally, and spiritually.

The key with exercise is consistency. Exercise at least three times a week. Start out with five minutes and then build on from there.

Read I Tim 4:8: What is more valuable than physical exercise? (p. 279)

SCRIPTURE MEMORY (P. 280)

Another discipline that you have learned about is scripture memory. It is thought that Paul had at least the first 5 books of the Bible memorized and likely had much more than that committed to memory

Share a verse you have memorized and its significance to you? (p. 281)

Have you considered memorizing verses, chapters, or books?

Scripture memory is frequently overlooked in busy schedules. See if the group will commit to memorizing some verses before next week. For some the thought of memorizing a chapter is too overwhelming. Encourage them to look at Psalm 117. This chapter is 2 verses long and each verse is rather short. Here is one chapter that is easy to memorize and this accomplishment may unlock the mental block against committing to memory whole chapters of God's Word. Continue this challenge even after class ends to encourage each other to set a goal of memorizing at least 4 scriptures per year.

TASTE AND SEE

Enjoy the good foods the class members brought in. Praise them for their contribution.

◆ ◆ ◆

VIDEO: We Were Made to Move

    View guide answer to Fill-ins:

    Ownership

    Occupancy

    Obedience

◆ ◆ ◆

WRAP IT UP

HOMEWORK

Read Week 12, *The Fullness of Christ,* and page 313 in the *Nutrition Manual.*

Banquet – Remind them to bring in their dish for the banquet next week. Decorate tables in the theme of the treasure hunt, have water available, encourage participants to invite guests – spouse, friends, church staff, etc. Ask someone to take pictures next week and then post on the group's Facebook page or church website. Send pictures to the Designed Healthy Living Facebook, also.

NEXT WEEK'S TOPIC TEASER: *Never, Never, Never Give Up*

CLOSE IN PRAYER.

Week Twelve

The Fullness of Christ and Health — Never Give Up

AGENDA

(adjust the plan to fit your schedule – this is a suggested schedule)

> Welcome
>
> Prayer and Praise
>
> Review: Previous Weeks – Jeopardy (20 minutes)
>
> Video: Final Intro – Dr. Couey (3 minutes)
>
> Review: The Fullness of Christ (20 minutes)
>
> Video: "Never, Never, Never Give Up" (34 minutes)
>
> Video: Finale (3 minutes)
>
> Foodie Feast - Finale Banquet

BRING

- All items needed for banquet
- DVD 7
- Jeopardy Game Handouts – See Appendix

This is the most important chapter. As the leader pray for each person as they read the plan of salvation.

NOTE: This is your last week as the official leader of this class but this is just the beginning of your role as leader on this journey. Come this week with a smile on your face and a glad heart. Congratulations, you made it through 13 weeks. I am sure you have received numerous blessings along this journey and I know you worked long hours to make your class a success. May God richly bless you for all you have done to make this class possible and for all the lives you have touched.

Enjoy the banquet – don't miss the DVD session and most of all – RELAX.

I hope we meet someday to share a hug for all you have done on this journey together and to bring your friends along. It has been my joy to be praying for you.

Blessings to you,
Annette Reeder

WELCOME

PRAYER AND PRAISE TICKLES

REVIEW:

> On page 293 the treasure clue states: *Whatever you do in word or deed, do all in the name of the Lord Jesus, giving thanks through Him to God the Father.* Colossians 3:17

> What is left out in this verse?

> Does it include shopping, cooking, our jobs, or our relationship with our neighbors?
>> *So this means nothing is left out.*

> Do we ever say "whatever" to God? Do we really mean "I surrender all?"

THANKFULNESS

> Who would like to share the four things God brought to your mind from this class for which you are thankful? (p. 295)
>> *Give them a chance to respond. Don't rush the Holy Spirit.*

> How can we teach our family to be thankful?

Being thankful for the foods God has given us will help us value these foods above man's innovations that turn out to be void of nutrition and fiber.

LAUGH AND LIVE LONGER

> What happens in our protein membrane when we experience laughter?
>> *They are wide open – able to let nutrients in and toxins out.*

> What are the benefits of joy in our life?
>> *Own answers.*

SHARE:

I would like to share with you the words of Oswald Chambers and his view of abundant joy from 2 Corinthians 7:4 – "The undiminished radiance which is the result of abundant joy is not built on anything passing but on the love of God that nothing can change. And experiences of life, whether they are everyday events or terrifying ones are powerless to separate us from the love of God which is in Christ Jesus our Lord."

For those of you who read the Wordless Book and found this was the first time you truly understood God's plan for you, which includes the gift of salvation, please come and share it with me or go and share with your pastor. Salvation is truly the ultimate treasure you will ever find and it is one that will carry you through this life on eagle's wings.

ACTION PLAN AND RESULTS OF MY HUNT

Let's celebrate the conclusion and look at your Action Plan. Review *Results of My Hunt* on page 235 and *Health Assessment* on page 233. The *Results of My Hunt* will be a good checklist of all the changes each participant has made. Many times people take this class and feel too overwhelmed to think they can ever do anything right. But by checking off the items or changes they have already made is a confirmation that they actually can do this – just never give up.

After reviewing the Action Plan, Results of My Hunt and the Health Assessment, let them share Praise Tickles.

JEOPARDY – This game was put together from the Teacher Manual for leading children of all ages through this journey. Have fun with it. Here are the questions by category.

Treasure of Health

100 Points

A. Receive His Word, treasure His commandments, discover the knowledge of God

Q. What are the three main things God wants us to do?

200 Points

A. Wisdom, knowledge, and understanding

Q. What God will give us in return for our obedience?

300 Points

A. Measuring men's words and advice and measuring them against the Bible, and putting those things into practice that match up with God's Word.

Q. What does it mean to be wise?

400 Points

A. To protect us, benefit us, and draw us into closer fellowship with Him.

Q. Why does God give us laws and rules to live by?

500 Points

A. (1)Eat only substances God created for food. Avoid what is not designed for food. (2)As much as possible, eat foods as they were created – before they are changed or converted into something humans think might be better.

(3) Avoid food addictions. Don't let any food become your god.

Q. What are The Three Principles?

Beverages

100 Points

A. Jesus is essential for spiritual life and water is essential for physical life.

Q. Why are both Jesus and water important?

200 Points

A. Fatigue, flushed skin, headache, infrequent and dark yellow urine, dizziness, loss of appetite, muscle cramps, etc.

Q. What are some signs of dehydration?

300 Points

A. It provides protein, lactoferrin, carbohydrates, healthy fats, water and fat soluble vitamins, minerals, enzymes, and beneficial bacteria.

Q. What makes milk a power food?/ What is milk?

400 Points

A. It inhibits growth of cancer cells, kills cancer cells without harming healthy tissue, lowers LDL (bad) cholesterol, and inhibits the abnormal formation of blood clots.

Q. What are the benefits of green tea?/ What is green tea?

500 Points

A. Thin drinks are 10 calories per ounce and thick drinks are 20 calories per ounce.

Q. How can we calculate the calories in the things we drink?

Grains

200 Points

A. 1 – Grains, nuts, and seeds are all foods provided by God in plenty. 2 – Eating nuts and seeds in their raw state retains the most nutrients; milling your own flour keeps it closest to its natural state. 3 – Remember that grains are an important part of nutrition, but Jesus is the bread of life and we should always crave Him more than any food.

Q. How can the Three Principles be applied to grains, nuts, and seeds?

400 Points

A. Grains can easily grow all over the world; grains have a long shelf life; the variety of grains available and nutrition found in them

Q. How do grains provide evidence of a creator?

600 Points

A. It provides energy, helps control weight, and aids in disease prevention

Q. Why is fiber important?/What is fiber?

800 Points

A. Heart healthy, prevention of free radical damage, slows aging, helps maintain healthy cell membranes

Q. What are the top benefits of Vitamin E?/What is Vitamin E?

1000 Points

A. Jesus, who is the bread of life and essential for eternal life

Q. What is the most important symbol bread represents?

Vegetables & Fruits

200 Points

A. Broccoli, Kohlrabi, Cauliflower, Kale, Turnip, Radishes, Rutabaga, Cabbage, Watercress, Brussels Sprouts, Mustard Greens, & Horseradish.

Q. What are cruciferous vegetables?

400 Points

A. Make up your mind

Q. What is one of the most important things to do in order to be able to stick with healthy eating?

600 Points

A. Follow guidelines in labeling and make food the most enticing to purchase.

Q. What are the manufacturer, producer, and seller's purposes behind food labels and stickers?

800 Points

A. Community Supported Agriculture - an opportunity for individuals and families to join in a farm venture as a member or shareholder

Q. What is a CSA?

1000 Points

A. sight, smell, taste, and touch

Q. What senses should we use when picking produce?

Herbs, Spices, Oil, & Vinegar

200 Points

A. Frankincense; myrrh; gall; mustard; hyssop; wormwood

Q. What different herbs are listed in the Bible?

400 Points

A. They were used to help bring to the Israelites memory the suffering they experienced in Egypt and God's miraculous delivery from slavery.

Q. What was the purpose of bitter herbs during Passover?

600 Points

A. They help digestion, the liver filter harmful substances, the metabolism of fat, managing blood-sugar problems, and reverse stomach ulcers

Q. What health benefits do bitter herbs provide?

800 Points

A. If we are confrontational or legalistic about how we present the gospel, it becomes impalatable.

Q. How can we be "too salty" in our speech?

1000 Points

A. Relieves chronic fatigue, relieves headaches, improves digestion, combats mucus, rids the body of toxins, strengthens the heart, fights kidney and bladder problems, and helps prevent constipation.

Q. What are the benefits of cooking and eating with vinegar?

Protein & Meat

100 Points

A. It provides the structure for all living things; is a necessary part of every living cell in the body; makes up muscles, ligaments, tendons, organs, glands, nails, hair, hormones, and many vital organs; is needed for vitamins and minerals to be absorbed and assimilated; provides energy directly to muscles.

Q. What is Protein?

200 Points

A. It reduces plaque that clogs arteries, blood clots, and blood vessel spasms.

Q. What are Omega-3 oils?

300 Points

A. Where a chicken has been raised and what it has eaten.

Q. What determines the nutritional value of an egg?

400 Points

A. The law was a shadow of the promise of the new covenant between God and people. Jesus came to fulfill God's law, obeying it complete, in a way that we cannot.

Q. What does it mean that Jesus came to fulfill the law?

500 Points

A. 2 each of the unclean and 7 each of the clean

Q. How many animals did Noah bring on the Ark?

Fasting & Self-Discipline

200 Points

A. A means to worship the Lord and submit ourselves in humility to Him.

Q. What is fasting?

400 Points

A. Abstaining from food, completely or partially, for a specified period of time.

Q. How is fasting defined?

600 Points

A. We live in a feel-good society and don't want to be bothered with any thought of hunger and self-denial.

Q. Why do most people avoid fasting?

800 Points

A. Normal; Absolute; & Partial

Q. What are the three types of fasting?

1000 Points

A. Disciplining our bodies to do what is best and in line with God's perfect will, rather than allowing our bodies, desires, and feelings to lead our actions.

Q. What is self-control?

Sweets

100 Points

A. It contains vitamins, minerals, enzymes and amino acids.

Q. What are some of the benefits of honey?/ What is honey?

200 Points

A. It actually drains nutrients from your body.

Q. What is an anti-nutrient?

300 Points

A. Depressed immunity; negative impact on behavior, attention and learning; increased obesity; increases sugar highs, promotes diabetes and heart disease; mal-nutrition and cavities; osteoporosis; increased yeast problems, and acceleration of the aging process.

Q. What can happen to our bodies when we eat too much sugar?

400 Points

A. They increase appetites in general and interfere with taste, enjoyment and satisfaction obtained from eating foods high in complex carbohydrates.

Q. What are artificial sweeteners?

500 Points

A. 5 pounds per year!

Q. How much sugar do you think the average American ate in the 1700's?

Environment & Toxins

200 Points

A. He sought the Lord and declared a fast.

Q. What did King Jehoshaphat do when threatened by invaders?

400 Points

A. Liver.

Q. What is our body's most important defense against toxins?

600 Points

A. Household cleaners.

Q. What is the most frequent contributing source of toxic chemicals in our lives?

800 Points

A. A very fine, slightly acidic film on the surface of our skin acting as a barrier to bacteria, viruses, and other potential contaminants that may penetrate the skin.

Q. What is the acid mantle?

1000 Points

A. Our Skin.

Q. What is our body's largest organ?

Stress & Forgiveness

100 Points

A. Environment, diet, lack of exercise and attitude.

Q. What are the four main causes of stress?

200 Points

A. Scripture – read it, study it, meditate on it, and memorize it.

Q. What's the best way to develop a positive attitude?

300 Points

A. To distract us and keep our focus off God.

Q. How does Satan use stress?

400 Points

A. To teach us to fully depend and rely on Him.

Q. How does God use stress?

500 Points

A. It is like carrying around extra weight. It can cause achy joints, heart rate increases, tight muscles, headaches, and upset stomachs.

Q. What is un-forgiveness?

If time permits before showing the video, this quote would be good to share with the class:

> **Future Foods**
>
> 'Nature' has elegantly designed foods to provide us with a complex array of dozens of nutrients and thousands of additional compounds that may benefit health—most of which we have yet to identify or understand. Over the years, man has deconstructed food and then reconstructed them in an effort to "improve" them. With new scientific understandings of how nutrients—and the myriad of other compounds in foods interact with genes, we may someday be able to design foods to meet the exact health needs of each

individual. Indeed, our knowledge of the human genome and of human nutrition may well merge to allow for specific recommendations for individuals based on their predisposition to diet-related diseases. If the present trend continues then someday physicians may be able to prescribe the perfect foods to enhance your health. And farmers will be able to grow them. Scientists have already developed gene technology to alter the composition of food crops. They can grow rice enriched with vitamin A and tomatoes containing a hepatitis vaccine, for example. It seems quite likely that foods can be created to meet every possible human need. (*Understanding Normal and Clinical Nutrition*, 7th Edition, 2006, Thomson Learning, p 469)

Because man will always try to improve on God's design for greed or other reasons we need to learn to never give up on God's perfect plan.

♦ ♦ ♦

VIDEO: "Never, Never, Never Give Up"

VIEWER GUIDE ANSWERS

Jeremiah 31:3 I have loved you with an <u>everlasting</u> love.

Philippians 4:19 He supplies <u>all</u> you need according to His riches in glory.

We have an opportunity to reach others with the <u>power</u> of food.

When scriptural principles are forgotten we become slaves to:

<u>Sugar, laziness,</u> processed food, self-centeredness, <u>unforgiveness</u> and obesity.

These are signs of us wanting to be in <u>charge</u>.

He who controls our food has the most <u>power</u>. He who has the <u>power</u> controls us.

Our fight is against <u>Satan</u>.

Does Satan want you to share this news? <u>NO</u>

Does God want you to share what you have been doing? <u>YES</u>

1 Corinthians 10:13

Galatians 6:9 And let us not lose heart in doing <u>good</u>, for in due time we shall reap if we do not grow weary.

If you view your body as a gift from God on loan then I ask you to never, never, never give up treating it like a <u>gift</u>.

♦ ♦ ♦

VIDEO: Finale

WRAP IT UP – Enjoy the banquet!

CLOSE IN PRAYER.

APPENDIX A

Student Handouts

These handouts are for students to use
along with the DVD/video presentations.

ARE YOU READY TO DISCOVER THE TREASURE OF HEALTH?

PSALM 34:8

Taste and see that the Lord is good, blessed is the man who trusts in Him.

Taste means: _____

See means: _____

DEFINE THE DESTINATION

Words that summarize the health you desire:

_____

_____

_____

GRAB YOUR GEAR

OUR MAP IS OUR MOST IMPORTANT PIECE OF GEAR.

PROVERBS 2:6

For the Lord gives _____; From His mouth comes _____ and _____.

PSALM 119:92-93

If your law had not been my delight, then I would have perished in my affliction. I will _____ Your precepts, for by them you have _____ me!

PROVERBS 3:7-8

Trust in the Lord with all your heart and do not lean on your own understanding. In all your ways acknowledge Him and He will make your paths straight. Do not be wise in your own eyes, fear the Lord and turn away from evil. It will be _____ to your body and _____ to your _____.

EXODUS 15:26

If you listen _____ to the voice of the Lord your God and _____ what is right in his eyes and _____ _____ to His commandments, and _____ all His statutes, I will put none of the diseases on you which I have put on the Egyptians, for I am the Lord _____ _____.

DEUTERONOMY 4:39-40

Know therefore _____, and take it to your heart that the Lord, _____ _____ _____ in heaven above and on the earth below; there is _____ other. So you shall keep His statutes and His commandments which I am giving you today that it may go well with you and with your _____ after you and that you may _____ _____ _____ _____ _____ which the Lord Your God is giving you for all time.

OUR COMPASS GIVES US DIRECTION

Your five favorite foods:

_____

_____

_____

_____

_____

THE THREE PRINCIPLES

Principle I: Eat only substances God created for food.

Principle II—Eat the foods as they were created - with very little alteration.

Principle III: Don't let any food become your god.

John Piper: What we _____ for, we _____.

Fasting is a very effective way of freeing ourselves from a preoccupation with our physical wants and desires so that we can concentrate on our relationship with God.

TAKE THE TREASURES

Foodie Friends

Health and food is our new approach to build relationships that lead to an opportunity for witnessing.

Reaching our final destination – acquiring the treasure of health outlined in the Bible will allow us to be balanced, wise, and healthy.

Are you ready to discover and experience the treasure?

Week One

$ HOW HEALTHY IS YOUR BANK ACCOUNT? $

I pray that in all respects you may prosper and be in good health. 3 John 1:2

DAILY CHOICES:

- ❑ Food & Water
- ❑ _____ foods build the _____ body.
- ❑ Whole Food Supplements
- ❑ Sleep
- ❑ Consumer Products

- ❑ Exercise
- ❑ Air
- ❑ Attitude & Focus on God

Healthy Savings Account Payout

- Better Resistance to _____
- Less or no _____ and _____
- Mental _____
- Energy and Flexibility (_____ and _____)
- Blood Sugar _____
- Look _____ Feel _____
- Great _____

HEALTH EXPENSES:

- ❑ _____ _____ Diet
- ❑ Sugar
- ❑ Synthetic _____
- ❑ Toxins
- ❑ _____ Mentality
- ❑ Lack of _____

- ❑ Dehydration
- ❑ _____ Exercise
- ❑ OTC and Rx _____
- ❑ Unforgiveness
- ❑ Stress

More health expenses than income = _____

Week One

MINDLESS EATING TO MINDFUL EATING

How long will you love what is worthless and aim at deception? Psalm 4:2

Factors contributing to our mindless eating

- ♦ _____
- ♦ _____
- ♦ TV
- ♦ _____
- ♦ Your _____
- ♦ Size of _____
- ♦ Size of _____ and Number of _____

ARE YOU REALLY HUNGRY?

Physical Hunger

- ♦ Builds _____
- ♦ Strikes _____ the neck
- ♦ Occurs _____ hours after a meal
- ♦ _____ when full
- ♦ Eating leads to feelings of _____

Emotional Hunger

- ♦ Develops _____
- ♦ _____ the neck
- ♦ Unrelated to _____
- ♦ _____ despite fullness
- ♦ Eating leads to _____
  and _____

Cues to the good stuff

- ♦ Be _____
- ♦ Think 20%
- ♦ Set a beautiful _____
- ♦ Be vigilant
- ♦ Keep your _____
- ♦ Watch your and your spouse's _____

- ♦ Experience the _____
- ♦ Eat _____
- ♦ Minimize _____
- ♦ Keep it simple
- ♦ Give thanks

You are the nutritional gatekeeper.

Gate keepers control _____ of the food decisions of their children and spouse.

Thou hast put gladness in my heart, more than when grain and new wine abound. Psalm 4:7

Week Two

IT'S A RADICAL LIFE

All living things begin as a _____.

A group of cells create a type of _____.

A group of tissues create a particular _____.

A group of organs create an _____.

A group of organ systems create an _____. Like You ☺.

Everything that happens in the body happens at the _____ _____.

Healthy cells = healthy tissues = healthy organs= healthy organ systems.

Unhealthy cells = unhealthy tissues = unhealthy organs= unhealthy organ systems

The human body has 11 organ systems, how many you can name?

_____

_____

_____

Our Bodies have trillions of cells. These cells continually work for you 24/7 and 365:

❑ _____
❑ _____
❑ _____
❑ _____
❑ _____

Basic needs of a cell:

❑ _____
❑ _____
❑ _____
❑ _____

Each person's responsibility:

1. Supply _____   2. Avoid _____

Free Radicals

Free radicals can be helpful:

- Produced in metabolism (this is a normal process – higher metabolism: more free radicals)
- Destroy viruses and bacteria
- Produce vital hormones
- Activate enzymes.
- Produce energy

Free radicals can be harmful:

- Damage cell membranes
- Attack the cell's DNA
- Contribute to aging.
- Contribute to abnormal cell growth
- Disrupt chemical reactions

Are they all Bad? _____

What contributes to free radicals?

- ❑ Processed Foods – The White Stuff
- ❑ Synthetics
- ❑ Chemicals
- ❑ Radiation
- ❑ Waste Products
- ❑ Additional sources: Caffeine, alcohol, soda, nicotine, unpurified water, rancid oils, nitrites, processed meats, synthetic vitamins, synthetic hormones, food flavorings, additives, preservatives, colors, household cleaners, air fresheners, personal care products, heavy metals: aluminum, mercury, lead, x-rays, cat scans, off-gassing from furniture and building materials, paint, carpet, plastics, new cars, dental work, root canals, metal fillings, plastic wrap, plastic toys, hair salons, plus much more, if you can believe it.

What can be done? **The Answer to Free Radical Damage:** _____

Antioxidants are God's gift for free radical "damage control".

1. Provide the extra _____.
2. Provide a _____ shield.
3. _____ the free radical

Where do we get natural antioxidants?

- Phytonutrients: found in fresh fruits, veggies, sprouts, green drinks, etc.,

- Beta carotene: works in both fat and water soluble areas interrupting the chain reaction. Beta-carotene is not destroyed after it immobilizes the free radical.

- Vitamin E works to protect the fat soluble areas and shield the cell from attack. Vitamin E is immobilized after a "hit".

- Vitamin C: works in water soluble areas and recharges vitamin E power after it disarms the free radical. Vitamin C detoxifies harmful free radicals.

- The minerals: zinc, selenium, copper, manganese, magnesium.

- Certain enzyme systems.

- Various herbs: bilberry, ginkgo biloba, Siberian ginseng, etc.

- Green tea: contains polyphenols. Your order of antioxidants and source is switched here.

How many do we require? _____

Week Three

It's a Radical Life – so live it wisely!

DIVINE DESIGN IN DIGESTION

Rhonda Sutton, RN, MSN

THE ORDER OF DIGESTION

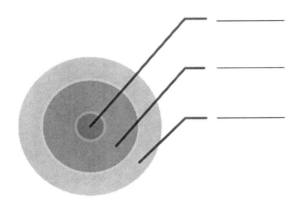

Our food choices are _____ to our health.

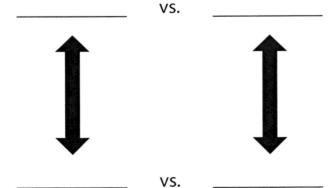

The digestive process is the center for _____ and _____.
Our choices determine energy for living or fatigue and illness.

The Flow of Digestion:

Elimination should happen _____ times per day.

To feel our best we _____

Most digestive problems we experience today come from four major sources:

_____ _____ choices

_____ _____ fiber

Too much _____

_____ Environment

The digestive tract can heal itself in 3-5 _____.

Constipation

The number one reason for constipation is lack of _____.

We need _____ grams of fiber per day.

Fiber:

- Increases the bulk of the stool
- Increases the size of the stool
- Acts like a magnet and pulls out toxins
- Cleans the colon

If fiber is not there to take out the toxins the body sends them to the _____ system.

Functions of the Immune System

Protects, Repairs and _____ Disease

Leaky Gut

Leaky Gut syndrome causes many illnesses such as arthritis, asthma, auto-immune disease, digestive problems (such as colitis, diverticulitis, IBS, etc.) fatigue, food allergies, chronic fatigue syndrome and fibromyalgia.

What restores normal function?

1. _____ & _____
2. _____

   These affect the body's ability to absorb nutrition and help maintain a healthy intestine.
3. Reduce _____

   Foods with a calming effect include herb teas, like chamomile. Deep breathing, exercise and relaxing activities help restore balance, peace of mind and joy for living.

4. Provide and Protect _____ and Vitamins

   Best source for enzymes are raw fruits and vegetables.

5. Resist Late Night and _____

   Our liver works for us to keep us healthy so we need to let it repair itself every night from 12 – 2 by not eating late and not eating too much.

Our food choices are not just a _____ matter but a _____ matter also.

Everything is permissible for me, but not everything is beneficial. 1 Corinthians 6:12

Week Four
GO FOR THE GOOD

Genesis 1:31

God saw _____ that He had made and behold it was _____

Good: _____

Valuable in estimation

❑ **DISCOVER THE GOOD: YOUR OWN BACKYARD**

❑ **DISCOVER THE GOOD: FARMERS MARKETS**

Questions to ask a local farmer:

What is your favorite pick of the day? Do you have anything unusual?

Does this produce come from your farm?

When did you pick this fruit or vegetable? Is it ready to eat today? How do I store it?

Do you use synthetic products like pesticides or fungicides?

Do you have a favorite recipe or way of preparing this vegetable?

Thank the farmer for his/her time.

❑ **DISCOVER THE GOOD: GROCERY STORE**

Fresh is best.

See the ***Tips for Picking Your Produce*** on the website: www.designedhealthyliving.com

Protect Our Produce

Store unwashed – wash immediately prior to use

Handle stone fruits properly – will continue to ripen after picking

Wash hands first then wash the produce

Long Term Storage

> Dried   Canned   Frozen

See the website for resources for Waterless Stainless Steel Cookware

and the Excalibur Dehydrator, www.designedhealthyliving.com

DON'T SETTLE FOR LESS THAN THE GOOD!

Week Five

MAKING MELODY WITH OUR HEARTS

Speaking to one another in psalms, and hymns and spiritual songs, singing and making melody with your heart to the Lord. Ephesians 5:19

CPR: _____, _____ and _____

Let's _____ to be _____

Exodus 23:2 Do not follow the crowd in doing wrong.

3 John 11: Do not imitate what is evil but what is good.

CARE

Herbs

Garlic

PROTECT – HOW CAN WE PROTECT OUR HEART?

Cardiovascular Disease is always one of the top causes of death in America

5 factors that cause insult or injury to the lining of the artery:

1.

2.

3.

4.

5.

_____% of those who suffer a heart attack never live to tell about it.

Hosea 4:6 My people perish from lack of knowledge.

Other contributors to heart disease or advancing the disease: (see page 234-235 in Nutrition Manual)

Improper diet	Smoking
Stress	Other health concerns
Lack of exercise and overweight	

<u>Diet</u> – body needs healthy fat. – Olive Oil (page 76 in Nutrition Manual)

Fats help our bodies in these ways:

Hormones	Cell membranes
Brain development	Energy

Healthy skin   Inflammation

Vasodilation

_____ fats are very necessary.

Some fats _____ and others _____

REVITALIZE

5 steps to revitalizing your heart:

1. Aspirin
2. Stay at normal weight and exercise
3. Lower fat in diet
4. Eat more fiber
5. Get adequate amounts of nutrients

   Calcium/ magnesium – regulates heartbeat, reduces hypertension

   Vitamin E – Decreases platelets clumping, decreases oxidation of fatty acids, dilates blood vessels, increases oxygen available to muscles and tissues, increase energy levels, may keep injury from ever happening, reverses plaque build-up and increases HDL.

   Vitamin C – Improves elasticity of blood vessels, builds capillary strength, antioxidant, builds red blood cells, helps protect other nutrients.

   Omega 3, EPA, GLA – Reduces triglycerides, reduces cholesterol, lowers hypertension, prevents blood clots, and reduces platelet stickiness, slippery blood vessels.

   B Complex – Low homocysteine, needed to deal with stress.

   Protein – strengthens heart muscle, forms healthy blood cells

   Fiber – Soluble fiber binds with cho9lesterol and keeps it from being reabsorbed, lowers cholesterol, improves digestion and elimination.

"There's within my heart a melody; Jesus whispers sweet and low' 'Fear not I am with thee peace, be still,' In all of life's ebb and flow." *He Keeps Me Singing,* Luther B. Bridgers

Week Six

WE HAVE A PROBLEM: INFLAMMATION

Dr. Richard Couey

God's creation of the cell: We have 100 trillion cells.

God made our body out of _____ chemicals.

_____ chemical reactions per second

There are approximately _____ in the human cell.

6 THINGS THAT CONTROL YOUR CHEMISTRY:

Three basic cell requirements:

1. _____ - cells getting the proper amount of the 27 chemicals.
2. _____ - to create energy we must exercise – therefore increase oxygen
3. _____ _____
    A. Limit Saturated fat
    B. Exercise
    C. Hydrate

Attitudes also affected your body chemistry

4. Mental
5. Emotional
6. Spiritual attitudes also affect your _____ _____.

We are a 4 part person: physical, mental, emotional and spiritual.

Protein membranes:

❑   ❑

❑   ❑

❑   ❑

Inflammation: What is it? (See *Treasures of Health Nutrition Manual* (pp. 219-225) for more information)

What shouldn't I eat? – see the Nutrition Manual for answers

What should I eat? – see the Nutrition Manual for answers

Why are Americans, specifically Christians, so sick? We are lazy

Week Seven

FOUR STEPS TO SELF-CONTROL

Like a city that is broken into and without walls is a man who has not control over his spirit.
Proverbs 25:28 (A city without walls is a disgrace because that is their protection.)

RECOGNIZE OUT OF CONTROL – DISTRACTIONS

A – Appetite – Proverbs 13:25

B- Brain

    MSG

    Aspartame

    Other Chemicals

C- Counterfeits – James 1:17

    John 10:10

RECOGNIZE WHOSE WE ARE – DISCIPLES

    Genesis 1:26

Lies People Believe

❑ **Lie #1 –I AM MY BODY**

1 Samuel 16:7 – *for God sees not as man sees, for man looks at the outward appearance but the Lord looks at the heart*

❑ **Lie # 2—I CANNOT CHANGE**

Isaiah 40:29 – *He gives strength to the weary, and to him who lacks might He increases power.*

❑ Lie # 3 –I'LL NEVER BE GOOD ENOUGH

Psalm 34: 4 – *I sought the Lord and He answered me and delivered me from all my fears.*

❑ Lie # 4 –I'M ALL ALONE

1 John 4:12 — *By this we know that we abide in Him and He in us because He has given us of His spirit.*
Proverbs 8:17— *I love those who love me*

❑ Lie # 5 –I CAN'T FORGIVE MY SELF

Acts 26:18 Paul's testimony where he quotes Jesus: *I am sending you to open their eyes so that they may turn from darkens to light and from dominion of Satan to God in order that they may receive forgiveness of sins and an inheritance among those who have been sanctified by faith in me.*

RECOGNIZE THE NEED FOR CHANGE – DISCERNMENT

If you have the faith of a mustard seed you shall say to this mountain, move from here to there and it shall move and nothing shall be impossible. Matthew 17:20

Getting started with discernment:
1. Repent of this problem
2. Pray about fasting
3. Journal every day
4. Design an eating plan
5. Pick a time to get started
6. Choose a Bible verse to meditate on daily

RECOGNIZE GOD'S PLAN – DELIVERANCE

If a man cleanses himself from these things he will be a vessel for honor, sanctified, useful to the Master, prepared for every good work. 2 Timothy 2:21

OVERCOMING COMPULSIVE OVEREATING

DON'T BELIEVE THESE LIES:

- ❏ **Lie #1 – I AM MY BODY**

  Some believe they are their bodies and that they will not be acceptable and worthwhile until their bodies carry less weight. 1 Samuel 16:7

- ❏ **Lie # 2 – I CANNOT CHANGE**

  Some feel powerless and out of control about food, their bodies, themselves and their potential to change. Isaiah 40:29

- ❏ **Lie # 3 – I WILL BEVER BE GOOD ENOUGH**

  Some never feel good enough, smart enough, responsible enough or perfect enough. Psalm 34:4

- ❏ **Lie # 4 – I AM ALL ALONE**

  Some feel alone, unlovable or feel discounted. 1 John 4:12, Proverbs 8:17

- ❏ **Lie #5 – I CANNOT FORGIVE MYSELF.**

  Some feel unable to forgive themselves for overeating. Acts 26:18

RECOVERY IS A PROCESS NOT A QUICK FIX.

Healing comes by being able to give healthy responses to questions such as:

Who am I?

What are my own thoughts, ideas, values and feelings? (Compulsive overeaters are typically people pleasers – not able to voice their own opinions)

What are my own wants and needs?

What scares me, angers me, pleases me, or saddens me?

What can I do when I feel fear, anger, joy, or sorrow besides when I eat?

How can I stop obsessive thoughts and compulsions to eat?

What stresses me and makes me tense?

What can I do when I feel tense and stressed besides eating mindlessly?

How can I ask others for what I need and want?

How can I learn to accept that I have a right to ask for about what I need and want?

How can I learn not to abandon myself all the time for the sake of others?

How can I learn to accept myself and be patient and harmless with myself as I heal?

How can I learn to forgive myself?

It is hard work to overcome overeating but with hard work it can happen and lead to a life that is free and fulfilling. It is like coming home.

Each day you must intentionally decide to trust God for deliverance, to trust yourself, to accept yourself, and to nourish yourself.

This will allow you to break free from compulsive overeating by learning to eat what you need and trusting yourself to make healthy choices and healthy proportions.

Recovery from an eating disorder is probably the most difficult task you will ever face. At times, it may seem impossible to you. Recovery demands every resource and every bit of courage you can muster.

Unfortunately, wanting to get better is not enough. You must change both your mind-set and your behavior; one without the other is not enough. And you must face the substance that represents so much to you and frightens you the most: food.

12 STEPS TO RECOVERY

1. Admit it – eating and thought of eating are out of control
2. Believe 2 things – change is possible and "I deserve to have a better life."
3. Make a decision to change. Decide to tolerate whatever feelings come up.
4. Inventory problems needing to be addressed. Write down symptoms: how you eat, how you exercise, how you punish yourself for eating, how you try to lose weight, how you degrade and criticize yourself and try to be perfect.
5. Share your inventory from number 4 with someone who can help.
6. Develop a plan – keep it simple. Include attainable goals – not overly ambitious nor complicated. Identify one problem at a time and work on it.
7. Fake it till you make it! Believe you are going to feel better. It may take a long time but believe anyway. Anxiety will disappear, obsessing over it or avoiding change only makes it worse.
8. Take life one day at a time or one meal at a time. If you have get into trouble, start again. Give yourself another chance. Very few people climb straight up a mountain.
9. Build in some rewards for your efforts. Recovery is hard work. Find ways to soothe yourself. List rewards and allow yourself one every day.

10. Talk about how you feel as you make changes. As you change your behavior more feelings will surface. To understand these feelings talk, talk, talk, write, write, and write in your journal.

11. Keep on changing. Each week review inventory and decide which one to attack next.

12. Believe in yourself and give yourself credit for a job well done.

SAMPLE PLAN – 10 POINT CONTRACT.

Give yourself one point daily for each item you complete. Strive for a 10 point day – it is more important than the weight on the scale. This is just a sample – use these ideas to design your own contract that meets your specific needs.

My Personal Contract for Success

PHYSICALLY- I will:

1. Journal my feelings.
2. Do something that feels good and is healthy every day.
3. Eat at the table every meal and snack – no eating on the couch, in the bedroom, at the computer or while playing games.
4. Eat at healthy times of the day and stick to these times.
5. Exercise daily.

MENTALLY – I will repeat these statements to myself a minimum of 5 times each daily.

1. I can do this with God.
2. I love my body – just as it is.
3. I love the Lord and He created me in His image.
4. Change is possible.
5. I deserve a healthy mind.

Suggested Supplements:

Whole food multi- vitamin

Protein – High quality soy protein powder (must be non-GMO, water processed)

B- Complex – extra is needed to overcome sugar cravings and mood swings

Vitamin C – in addition to the multi vitamin

Vitamin E – in addition to the multi vitamin

Zinc

Omega 3 fish oil

Alfalfa tablets

Herbs – Milk Thistle, and a combination of: magnesium, zinc, chromium, taurine, vanadium, alpha lipoic acid, and banaba leaf extract

*Dalton, Sharon; Overweight and Weight Management; Jane Hirschmann & Carol Munter, Overcoming Overeating; Eating Disorders, Raymond Lemberg.

Week Eight

SOLUTIONS FOR OUR IMMUNE SYSTEM

Ellie Cullen, RN

SUGAR AND THE IMMUNE SYSTEM

The immune system protects the body from foreign substances like heavy metals such as _____, _____ and arsenic. And pathogenic organisms like bacteria, virus and parasites.

Parts of the Immune System include: Thymus

White Blood Cells (T Cells)

Bone Marrow (Red Blood Cells)

Nasal Hairs

Skin

Pancreas, kidneys, liver, and thyroid

Lymphatic system

   Tonsils

Circulatory system

If the immune system is working correctly it can keep up with offending material and there is no overload.

Overload leads to _____

Antioxidants

Such as C and E, also included: Glutathione

Glutathione acts as a major _____

_____ can severely reduce or kill the very nutrients needed to make glutathione.

_____ is the number one enemy of the immune system.

Vitamins and Minerals-- critical to having healthy organs and a healthy immune system:

A, B, C, D, E, and the minerals _____ and _____

Omega 3 fatty acids

Magnesium

SOD – Super Oxide dismutase

Resveratrol

Nutriferon

Selenium

Pumpkin seed

Probiotics

Organic iodine

The thyroid cleans the blood every _____ minutes.

Essential Foods:

Organic fruits and vegetables

Protein – organic meats and chemical free protein powders

Whole Grains – such as freshly milled wheat

Vitamin B

Vitamin C

Vitamin D- 17 different cancers are linked to lack of vitamin D

Vitamin E (400 IU before getting an x-ray or airport x-rays)

Zinc (stress destroys zinc)

Iron

One food that will undermine all these efforts - _____

Sugar is the number one enemy of the _____

Role of the Pancreas: Produces insulin in response to stress and sugar; produces enzymes

Sugar:

Increases Insulin – thereby causing problems with the pancreas

Attracts yeast

Destroys B vitamin

Digestive Problems- weight gain, gas and bloating

It is imperative to prevent disease. And if disease does happen we need to find it in the earliest stages.

Proper blood testing gives us an advantage to prevention and early treatment, which could mean more years enjoying our family and being on mission for God.

Ellie Cullen, RN, Founder: Your Future Health; www.yourfuturehealth.com

Week Nine

PROTECTION: INCREASING OUR PERSONAL VALUE

(2 Part Series)

Top Ten Tips to De-Tox (Part 1)

1. Choose better body care products.
    CosmeticsDatabase.com.
    Avoid triclosan, BHA, fragrances, and oxybenzone.
    Choose: "pH balanced" and organic

2. Go organic & eat fresh foods.

3. Avoid fire retardants.
    PBDE

4. Pick plastics carefully.
    BPA
    Avoid clear, hard plastic bottles marked with a "7" or "PC"
    Stay away from toys marked with a "3" or "PVC."

5. Filter your tap water.

6. Wash your hands.
    www.bottlesandfoamers.com

7. Skip non-stick.

8. Use a HEPA-filter vacuum.

9. Use green organic cleaners & avoid pesticides.

10. Eat good fats and fresh milled high fiber bread.

We will stand before this house .... 2 Chronicles 20:9

For more information check out these resources:

www.designedhealthyliving.com – waterless-stainless steel cookware, household cleaner, bread making supplies

www.epa.gov

http://householdproducts.nlm.nih.gov

www.ewg.org

www.designedhealthyliving.com/resources

www.greengoeswitheverything.com

Green Goes With Everything, by Sloan Barnett, Atria Books, 2008.

INCREASING OUR PERSONAL VALUE Part 2

_____ that a man achieves or fails to achieve is a direct result of his _____.
— John Maxwell

DON'T MUTTER, DECLUTTER!

Established means – _____ or grow _____
1 Corinthians 15:10

Oswald Chambers: _The way we continually talk about our own inabilities is an insult to our Creator. To complain over our incompetence is to accuse God false of having overlooked us._

Christian, for good health to occur we must realize what we think, how our emotions affect us, and our belief in God, all play a significant role in making us healthy.
Dr. Dick Couey

Top four phrases that people typically say to themselves.

   1.

   2.

   3.

   4.

Our self-talk affects our _____.

Our thoughts can be:

Accurate   Inaccurate

Constructive   Destructive

Right   Wrong

Negative Self-Talk can:
   ❑ Limit hours of productivity
   ❑ Strain our relationships
   ❑ Inhibit our mental and emotional growth potential
   ❑ Increase stress
   ❑ Prevent forgiveness
   ❑ Causes immunity dysfunction

Positive Self-Talk can:
   ❑ Helps us reach our goals beyond our dreams

- ❑ Repair relationships
- ❑ Relieves stress
- ❑ Allow forgiveness
- ❑ Lowers stress hormones
- ❑ Increase immunity capability

Our state of mind affects the health of our _____.

FOUR TIPS TO DETOX OUR MIND

1. Think Differently – Turn negative thoughts into positive ones.

2. Take Thoughts Captive – Seek wisdom. James 1:5-6

3. Tune Into Thankfulness –A mind that is thankful has little room for negative thoughts. —Ephesians 5:20

4. Turn Truths Into a Treasure – Change our negative thoughts into a word from God.

Proverbs 31 - King James Version

Read each verse. Consider how the words can be personalized and turned into an affirmation. Write out this affirmation following each proverb.

Verse 10: Who can find a virtuous (righteous, honorable, good) woman? For her price is far above rubies.

NKJV – Who can find a virtuous wife? For her worth is far above rubies.

Example - I am an honorable wife; my desire is to be priceless in my husband's eyes.

Verse 11 - The heart of her husband doth safely trust in her, so that he shall have no need of spoil (no lack of gain).

NKJV – The heart of her husband safely trusts her; So he will have no lack of gain.

Example – My husband can trust me with the finances, home matters and training up our children. I continue to seek the best in each member of the family.

Verse 12 - She will do him good and not evil all the days of her life.

NKJV – She does him good and not evil all the days of her life. And willingly works with her hands.

Verse 13 - She seeketh wool, flax and worketh willingly with her hands.

NKJV – She seeks work and flax, and willingly works with her hands.

Verse 14 - She is like the merchant ships; she bringeth her food from afar.

NKJV – She is like the merchant ships, she brings her food from afar.

Verse 15 - She riseth also while it is yet night, and giveth meat to her household and a portion to her maidens.

She also rises while it is yet night, and provides food for her household and a portion for her maidservnats.

Verse 16 - She considereth a field and buyeth it; with the fruit of her hands she has planted a vineyard.

NKJV – She considers a field and buys it, from her profits she plants a vineyard.

Verse 17 - She girdeth her loins with strength and strengtheneth her arms.

NKJV – She girds herself with strength and strengthens her arms.

Verse 18 - She perceivieth that her merchandise is good; her candle goeth not out by night.

NKJV – She perceives that her merchandise is good, and her lamp does not go out by night.

Verse 20 - She stretches out her hand to the poor, yea; she reacheth forth her hands to the needy.

NKJV – She extends her hand to the poor, yes, she reaches out her hands to the needy.

Verse 21 - She is not afraid of the snow for her household; for all her household are clothed with scarlet.

NKJV – She is not afraid of snow for her household, for all her household is clothed with scarlet.

Verse 23 - Her husband is known in the gates, when he sitteth among the elders of the land.

NKJV – Her husband is known in the gates, when he sits among the elders of the land.

Verse 25 - Strength and honor are her clothing, and she shall rejoice in time to come.

NKJV – Strength and honor are her clothing, she shall rejoice in time to come.

Verse 26 - She opened her mouth with wisdom, and in her tongue is the law of kindness.

NKJV – She opens her mouth with wisdom, and on her tongue is the law of kindness.

Verse 27 – She watches over the ways of her household, and does not eat the bread of idleness.

Verse 28 - Her children rise up and call her blessed; her husband also, and he praiseth her.

NKJV – Her children rise up and call her blessed; her husband also, and he praises her.

Verses 29 – 31 - Many daughters have done virtuously, but those excellest them all. Favor is deceitful and beauty is vain, but a woman who feareth the Lord, she shall be praised. Give her the fruit of her hands and let her own works praise her in the gates.

NKJV – Many daughters have done well, but you excel them all. Charm is deceitful and beauty is passing, but a woman who fears the Lord, she shall be praised, Give her the fruit of her hands, and let her own works praise her in the gates.

Week Ten

FREEDOM FROM BITTERNESS

Jane Elder

Food was never the answer, but eating a lot of sweet foods made me feel better temporarily. I fought the cravings so hard, but I was focusing on the wrong thing. The bitterness was what I needed to get rid of.

Pray for those who abuse you, Luke 6:28.

For release from bitterness:

1. Where is the bitterness?
2. With God's help, forgive and let go.
3. Daily think about and pray for the person.
4. Speak positively when given the opportunity.

It didn't help because I had not given up my desire for revenge against this person.

New prayer:
"God, where did I fail you yesterday?
I confess what I have done wrong.
Please forgive me and cleanse me.
God, for this day, I choose to trust You.
I ask You for faith to trust You for today.
Lord, as I start this day, I choose hope.
Help me to be thankful throughout this day."

Trusting God to make things right in the end and letting go of desire for revenge brings good things:

- Calmness
- Peace
- Joy

Getting rid of bitterness brings light and freedom.

God can be trusted and He does want good for your life, despite the hurts we all experience. God will heal you, if you let Him.

THE HEALING POWER OF FORGIVENESS
Sue Becker

SUE'S BATTLE WITH CANCER

After 14 yrs. of dedicating their lives to teaching the benefits of healthy grains and colon health, Sue was diagnosed with colorectal cancer.

Now she began to question everything.

She asked God, "Have I ever heard from you — what is this all about?" But even in the middle of her question, she says that "God remained faithful.

But then her pastor called to tell her, "I am sure that you are doubting everything you have taught, but what you must remember, what you teach is truth. He also said that "we are to speak life unto death." The power of life and death is in our tongue.

UNFORGIVENESS

Jeremiah 17:9 - "the heart is _____ above all things, who can know it".

We deceive ourselves because we _____ things.

"My Own Dear Child ... I hear every whispered prayer you pray ... and if you unlock the door to your heart's hidden room, I will come in and dwell there, and bring the peace and the power of my Spirit with me". *Postcards*

BEHOLD I STAND AT THE DOOR AND KNOCK

Revelation 3:20

Doctors can deal with that tumor but only God can deal with your _____.

Closing questions:

Do you have a conflict in your heart?

What well in your heart have you allowed the enemy to stop up?

What door to a room in your heart have you locked?

2 Chronicles 7:14 — If my people, who are called by my name, will _____ themselves and pray, and turn from their wicked ways, then I will hear from heaven and heal their land.

WICKED WAYS OF THE CHURCH:

- Bitterness
- Unforgiveness
- Anger
- Gossip
- Slander
- Resentment
- Rejection

Recognize unforgiveness as your _____ _____.

1 John 1:9

Revelation 3:19-20.

As surely as you are _____ you are spiritual

As surely as you are _____ you are physical.

FREEDOM COMES TO THOSE WHO FORGIVE.

Week Eleven

WE WERE MADE TO MOVE

Dr. Richard Couey

I beseech you therefore, brethren, by the mercies of God, that you present your bodies a living sacrifice, holy, acceptable to God which is your reasonable service. Romans 12:1 (NKJV)

BENEFITS OF BEING PHYSICALLY FIT:
> Heart
>
> Blood
>
> Lungs
>
> Blood Vessels

Type of Exercise
> Cardiovascular training
>
> Muscular Strength
>
> Flexibility Exercise

Exercise Precautions
> Warm-up properly
>
> Doctor's clearance
>
> Dress properly
>
> Temperature awareness
>
> Wear proper shoes
>
> Stretching

How hard/often should we exercise?
> Intensity
>
> 220 – age = _____ - resting heart rate _____ =
>
> _____ x 60% = _____ + resting heart rate.

Duration

Homework for the rest of your life:
> Frequency

Why we as Christians should be fit:

- Jesus was fit
- Our bodies are God's greatest creation
- Scriptural principles
  - o_____
  - o_____
  - o_____

MAKING THIS PERSONAL

Write a personal program to follow this coming week:

Write a personal program to follow weeks 2 – 4

Write a personal commitment to exercise:

Christians should be the healthiest in the world; we have the best example in Jesus Christ.

Week Twelve

NEVER, NEVER, NEVER GIVE UP

Jeremiah 31:3 I have loved you with an _____ *love.*
This love includes giving us a design for our health.

Philippians 4:19 He supplied _____ *you need according to his riches in glory.*
We have an opportunity to reach others with the _____ of food.

NEVER GIVE UP BECAUSE SCRIPTURE IS OUR FOUNDATION
When scriptural principles are forgotten we become slaves to:

_____, _____, processed food, self-centeredness, _____
and obesity.

These are signs of us wanting to be in _____.

Galatians 5:1

Ezra 3:11

NEVER GIVE UP BECAUSE NOTHING CAN STEAL YOUR DREAM
Ezra 4:4-5

Examples of Distractions:

Water

Salt

Air

Grain

Ephesians 6:12

He who controls our food has the most _____ (on Earth). He has the _____
controls us.

Our fight is against _____

Ezra 4:12

Satan has much to lose when we get healthy following God's plan.

Does Satan want you to share this news? _____

Does God want you to share what you have been doing? _____

1 Corinthians 10:13

Galatians 6:9 And let us not lose heart in doing _____, *for in due time we shall reap if we do not grow weary.*

NEVER GIVE UP BECAUSE THE HOLY SPIRIT IS OUR GUIDE

Our body reports for duty every minute.

You report to duty every day to the Holy Spirit

A healthy body is useful to the Holy Spirit

How we view our body mirrors our world view.

If you view your body as a gift from God on loan then I ask you to never, never, never give up treating it like a _____. The treasure that it is.

Proverbs 4:20-22

Taste and See that the Lord is good, blessed is the man who trusts in him. Psalm 34:8

Fabulous Foodie Fun

Rutabaga   Kohlrabi   Parsnips

Turnips   Sweet potato   Fennel

Beets   Jicama   Leeks

1. _____ 2. _____

3. _____ 4. _____

5. _____ 6. _____

7. _____ 8. _____

9. _____

Fabulous Foodie Fun

Rutabaga   Turnips   Jicama

Kohlrabi   Beets   Fennel

Parsnips   Sweet potato   Leeks

1. _____ 2. _____

3. _____ 4. _____

5. _____ 6. _____

7. _____ 8. _____

9. _____

Stress & Forgiveness	Sweets	Protein & Meat	Beverages	Treasures of Health
100	100	100	100	100
200	200	200	200	200
300	300	300	300	300
400	400	400	400	400
500	500	500	500	500

Grains	Vegetables & Fruits	Herbs, Spices, Oil & Vinegar	Fasting & Self-discipline	Environment & Toxins
200	200	200	200	200
400	400	400	400	400
600	600	600	600	600
800	800	800	800	800
1000	1000	1000	1000	1000

Stress & Forgiveness	Sweets	Protein & Meat	Beverages	Treasures of Health
100	100	100	100	100
200	200	200	200	200
300	300	300	300	300
400	400	400	400	400
500	500	500	500	500

Grains	Vegetables & Fruits	Herbs, Spices, Oil & Vinegar	Fasting & Self-discipline	Environment & Toxins
200	200	200	200	200
400	400	400	400	400
600	600	600	600	600
800	800	800	800	800
1000	1000	1000	1000	1000

Treasures of Healthy Living

REGISTRATION FORM

Please Print!

Name: _____

Address:_____

_____

E-Mail Address: _____

Phone: _____ _____ _____

Class Location: _____

Time: _____ Facilitator: _____

- -

For Office use only: Fee:_____ Recvd. BS _____ NM _____ CB _____

Date Paid:_____   Amount: _____   Method: CC   Check   Cash

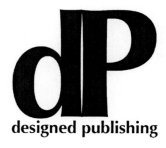
designed publishing

CPSIA information can be obtained at www.ICGtesting.com
Printed in the USA
BVOW050149070612

291990BV00006B/2/P